THEY WENT FROM FAT TO FABULOUS:

A DIET GUIDE FOR RESTAURANT LOVERS

by

E.S. Abramson

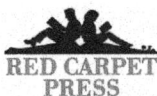

RED CARPET
PRESS

"Rolling Out the 'Read' Carpet, One Fantastic Book at a Time.™"

The information in this book reflects the author's experiences and opinions and is not intended to replace medical advice. Before beginning this or any nutritional or exercise program, consult with your physician to be sure it is appropriate for you.

ISBN-13: 9780692370872
ISBN-10:0692370870
LCCN: 2015945740

RED CARPET
PRESS

"Rolling Out the 'Read' Carpet, One Fantastic Book at a Time.™"
Red Carpet Press, L.L.C
P.O. Box 543
Hazelwood, MO 63042-0543
Red-Carpet-Press.com
Red@Red-Carpet-Press.com

Visit E. S. Abramson at:
www.ElaineAbramson.com
AAAuthor@aol.com

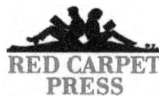

CITY OF ALBUQUERQUE

Office of the Mayor/ Chief Administrative Officer

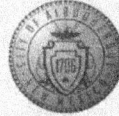

September 16th, 2013

Elaine Abramson
P.O. Box 16223
Albuquerque, NM 87191

Dear Ms. Abramson,

I wanted to congratulate you for the completion of your book From Fat to Fabulous: A Diet Guide for Restaurant Lovers. Your accomplishment of losing 85 pounds and 10 dress sizes while eating only restaurant meals is truly remarkable.

I find it extremely important to promote health and activity to the residents of Albuquerque. At the same time, our city is full of many wonderful restaurants, and enjoying dining out is not something that residents of the city should have to give up to maintain a healthy lifestyle. Your book will be very beneficial in educating the residents of the city on how to pick healthy, well-balanced and delicious meals while at the same time being able to enjoy socializing at their favorite dining establishments in the City of Albuquerque.

Congratulations again and I wish you continued good health and well-being.

Best regards,

Richard J. Berry
Mayor
City of Albuquerque

RJB: dm

PO Box 1293

Albuquerque

NM 87103

www.cabq.gov

Albuquerque - Making History 1706-2006

GOVERNOR OF MISSOURI

JEFFERSON CITY

65102

JEREMIAH W. (JAY) NIXON
GOVERNOR

P.O. Box 720
(573) 751-3222

October 7, 2013

Ms. Elaine Abramson
P.O. Box 543
Hazelwood, MO 63042

Dear Ms. Abramson:

It is my honor to congratulate you on the completion of your book *From Fat to Fabulous: A Diet Guide for Restaurant Lovers*. Your book is a great resource for those who enjoy dining out, while still maintaining a healthy lifestyle. Reducing obesity and diet-related diseases by promoting safe and healthy diets is a critical factor in improving the overall health of our citizens.

Again, congratulations and best wishes.

Sincerely,

Jeremiah W. (Jay) Nixon
Governor

BOOKS BY E. S. ABRAMSON

THURSDAY'S CHILD

ANOTHER THURSDAY'S CHILD

I AM THURSDAY'S CHILD

WE ARE THURSDAY'S CHILDREN

MARK OF KORESH

YESTERDAY'S MURDER

DAUGHTER OF SPIES

FROM FAT TO FABULOUS:
A DIET GUIDE FOR RESTAURANT LOVERS

THEY WENT FROM FAT TO FABULOUS:
A DIET GUIDE FOR RESTAURANT LOVERS

I would like to thank my fantastic husband Stan Abramson for all the time he spent editing, living with, and loving me as I went from *FAT TO FABULOUS*. He had so much faith in my diet that he went from *FAT TO FABULOUS* along with me.

CONTENTS

COVER PHOTOGRAPHS

<u>Top Center:</u> My husband Stan participates in the *From Fat to Fabulous Restaurant Lovers' Diet* along with me. Stan is wearing the size 22 vest I wore before I began the *Restaurant Lovers' Diet.*

<u>Lower Left and Lower Right:</u> Stan is wearing the size 22 blue coat I wore before I began the *From Fat to Fabulous Restaurant Lovers' Diet.*

In THURSDAY'S CHILD, a collection of forty-three short stories based on my life, the "Seventy-Five Cent Coat" story relates how I came to purchase the coat. I wore the coat for several years. After I went on my FAT TO FABULOUS RESTAURANT LOVERS' DIET, the coat hung on me. Now my husband wears the coat.

<u>Bottom Center:</u> The Inuit Indian extra-large sweater jacket I purchased in Toronto before I began my *From Fat to Fabulous Restaurant Lovers' Diet.*

TESTIMONIALS

"I've seen Elaine's restaurant diet in action - it's easy once you know what to do. And she looks great!" New York Times bestselling author Angie Fox.

"Your diet gives hope and shows that others can do it too." Ellie Searl, formatter of the first edition of FROM FAT TO FABULOUS: A DIET GUIDE FOR RESTAURANT LOVERS.

FROM FAT TO FABULOUS: A DIET GUIDE FOR RESTAURANT LOVERS is a great resource if you love to eat out (and who doesn't?) but need to know how to eat smart. Elaine Abramson has scored with this one! Judge Bill Hopkins, author.

"Second edition! Yeah! Your book has struck a chord!" Pam DeVoe, Anthropologist.

"Elaine Abramson proves you can lose weight and still eat out. She's a walking testament to smart eating by having the courage to ask for the right kind of food. FROM FAT TO FABULOUS: A DIET GUIDE FOR RESTAURANT LOVERS tells how she did it, so you can too! I highly recommend it." Sharon Woods Hopkins, author.

"I enjoyed the book. I am going to keep it in the car. Then when we go to different restaurants I can peek at the book and see what exchanges you made to make the meal a good one for us who are watching or trying to lose weight. Thanks again." Ruth Galayda.

FROM FAT TO FABULOUS

"There is no love more sincere than the love of food."
~ *George Bernard Shaw.*

WHEN PEOPLE ASK ME TO describe myself, I tell them "I have a body by disaster and hair by wash and beware". After God took one look at His creation, He trashed the mold. He didn't want to be responsible for creating another one like me. All kidding aside, immediately after I came into this world my mother had surgery for milk caking in her breasts - today doctors refer to it as cancer - and couldn't nurse me. I also developed an allergy to cow's milk. In the 1940's that left my mother with very few feeding options for me, so any nourishment I received was considered a blessing. But what was a blessing in the 1940's became a curse as the years passed. My body ballooned to proportions I was ashamed of; bathroom scales broke under my staggering weight.

After I lost eighty-five pounds on my *From Fat to Fabulous Restaurant Lovers' Diet* my husband was so proud of me he began telling people he'd lost a whole other wife.

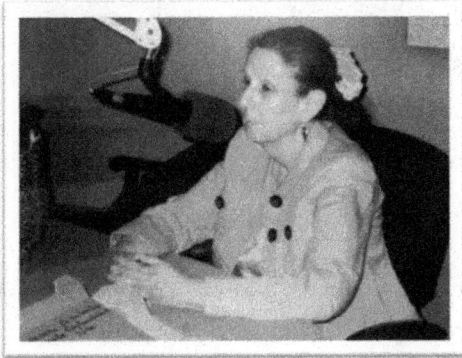

What surprised me the most was after I appeared on ABC and NBC TV in St. Louis, PBS in Cape Girardeau, and had my restaurant lovers' diet reviewed in the St. Louis Post-Dispatch health section and the

Riverfront Times dining out section, I received five marriage proposals. Ellie Searl, the woman who formatted the first *From Fat to Fabulous: A Diet Guide for Restaurant Lovers* for publication, said "Your diet gives hope and shows that others can do it too."

I am an award-winning artist and author, one lucky enough to have *Thursday's Child* and *Another Thursday's Child,* two collections of short stories based on my life, published. With credentials like that, you are probably asking what qualifies me to write another *From Fat To Fabulous: A Diet Guide for Restaurant Lovers.* I am a mother, grandmother, wife, and a woman who has spent her entire life fighting the battle of the bulge. My restaurant diet is the only diet on this earth that has ever worked for me. I have tried them all, only to gain the weight back on every one of them. But on my restaurant lovers' diet I went from a size 22 to a size 12 in one year and have enjoyed every minute of it. Now I am never hungry and have more energy than I have had during most of my life.

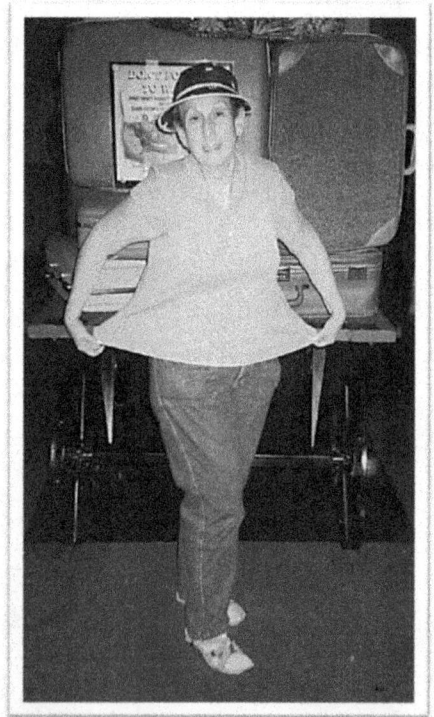

With the odds stacked against me, I lost 50 pounds in one year on my restaurant lovers' diet. During my second year on the diet I lost an additional 35 pounds. I have a sluggish thyroid, do not have a spleen, take medication that causes weight gain, had a slipped disk, and have bad knees which makes any form of exercise extremely difficult.

I have not prepared a meal in four years. The questions people ask most frequently about my diet are: 1) "Won't you get fat eating in restaurants?" Answer: not if you eat the right food. I tell them that by

eating only in restaurants I have gone from a size 22 to a size 12. 2) "Is it expensive to eat out?" My husband and I eat out Friday night, Saturday and Sunday lunch and dinner, and on special occasions. I clip coupons out of magazines and newspapers, print them off the Internet, and use them at restaurant chains and local independent establishments. Our favorite coupons are the buy-one-lunch-or-dinner and get-one-of-equal-value-free. Second to that were the thirty, twenty-five, and ten dollar off your total bill coupons. We do not buy entertainment or dining books because they never seem to have the restaurants we want to eat at.

One of the most over-looked restaurant bargains is the Early Bird special. It has become more and more popular at restaurants frequented by working people. DinnerBroker.com lists numerous restaurants that will take 30% off the bill if you eat there before 6 p.m. Some restaurants will also extend this discount throughout the evening. You make reservations on the restaurant's website and the discount is automatically applied to your bill. And 5pm.co.uk offers off-peak time restaurant discounts up to 50% in the United Kingdom.

My husband and I come home with so many take-out boxes that our refrigerator and freezer are always full. By using restaurant offers and coupons and by eliminating the fat I cut off meat and disposed of; olive or vegetable oil I dumped out after sautéing meat and vegetables; onion, potato and carrot peelings I threw in the garbage; meat and vegetable shrinkage during cooking; cost of using the stove and oven; cost of detergent and running the dishwasher; and all the other things I did to prepare a meal and clean up afterwards; there was only a slight difference in our food bills between what we spent in grocery stores

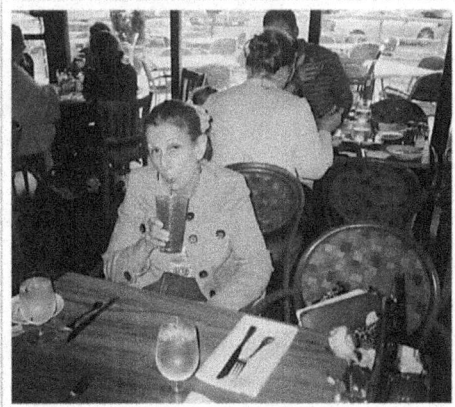

and what we spent in restaurants. Best of all, with all these leftovers, we have the convenience of not having to prepare a meal and the fun of choosing a different meal every time we eat.

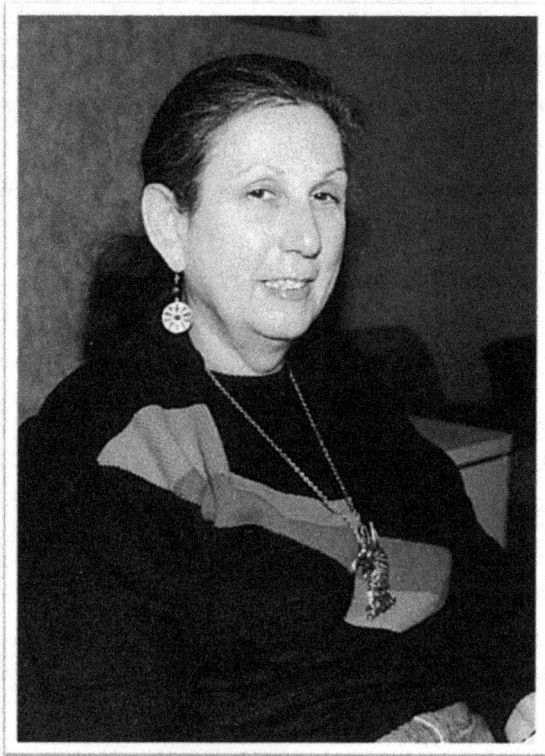

Long before I discovered my restaurant lovers, diet I bought the packaged, canned, and frozen foods required by weight loss programs and specific diets. They cost me far more than going out to restaurants ever did, and they did not help me lose weight, keep the weight off, or slim down. All I had were huge grocery bills and no results to show for it. I was always hungry after I ate the recommended portions, so I often found myself eating several portions to satisfy my hunger. Because these foods need to have grocery store shelf life, they are loaded with flour and wheat products, salt, sugar, and other preservatives, the very things that kept me fat.

I don't believe in fad diets, quick weight loss diets, or diets linked to support groups or diet groups where you must purchase the organization's food. I have failed at diets based on portion control, calorie counting, carb counting, weighing food, recording everything you eat in a diary, eating low fat or fat free foods, or any of the other numerous things that people who watch their weight do.

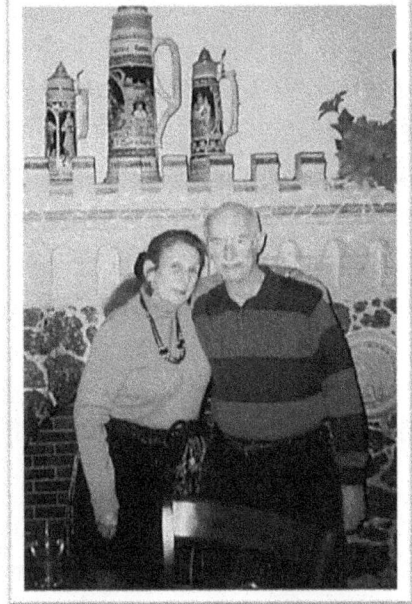

In an effort to slim down the population, the state of New York, several other states, and now the federal government require restaurants to publish calorie and other nutritional information on their menus. McDonalds, the largest fast food chain in the nation, was the first to post this information. But the restaurants that have already posted this information are finding out it does not work because most people tune out that information when placing their orders.

In an effort to attract people trying to lose weight, Longhorn has added a 550 calorie menu, Olive Garden a 575 calorie menu, Bravo!/Brio a 550 calorie menu, Mimi's Café has a 550 and under menu, and Subway a 5 grams of fat menu. Applebee's switched from the Atkins diet to 550 calorie meals. Colton's has a 700 calorie menu when paired with steamed veggies and using fat free dressing. IHOP has "Simple & Fit options", a list of what toppings, breads, syrups cheeses, and sugars to eliminate to have your dining choices contain less than 600 calories. While I applaud their efforts to help our obese population slim down, I would be bored limiting myself to just that small section of their menu, eating meals that eliminated the foods I like best, or eating at one restaurant over and over again.

Boredom is my enemy. It has doomed my past diets causing all of them to end in failure. I love my restaurant lovers' diet because I have endless choices of where to dine and almost endless choices of what I can eat. I eat at all of the restaurants I have mentioned, but I do not eat from their low calorie, fat free, or diet menus.

Olive Garden has a basket in the lobby filled with "Garden Fare Nutrition Guides." It lists the number of calories and the amount of fat, saturated fat,

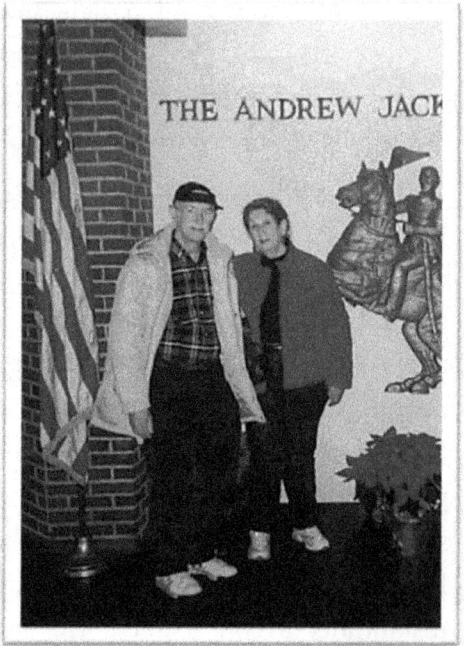

sodium, carbs, fiber, and protein in their meals, beverages, and desserts. I

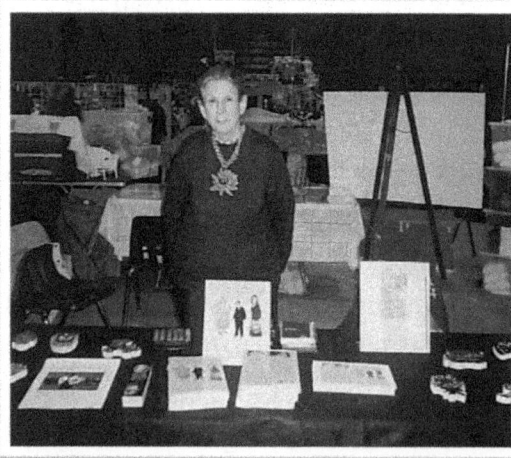

watched people hurry past the basket. Like me, they wanted to enjoy their food and not read a pamphlet that might make them feel guilty for eating the foods of their choice. Qdoba's and Wendy's "Nutrition" guides list calories, carbs, and fiber too. HuHot's "Allergy & Nutritional Information" also lists calories fat, fiber, and saturated fat. Qdoba's and HuHot's guides were left in their baskets, and ignored when diners placed their orders. IHOP's menu has photographs to tempt the palate. Like other IHOP diners, I too ignored the small squares at the top of the page listing "Under 600 Calories – Simple & Fit options" and ordered the foods I enjoy.

I read movie stars lose weight by eating grilled skinless chicken breasts, steamed vegetables, and vegetable salads without any dressing. Maybe they have more willpower than I have, but I could never stick to such a limited diet. It would bore me to death. Within days I would have reverted to my old eating habits and put on far more weight than I took off. I need a diet with infinite variety and one that also lets me make substitutions when necessary. I love my restaurant lovers' diet because it is *fun* and *easy* to follow.

Since going on my restaurant lovers' diet, I have not cooked a meal in over four years. If you are anything like me, cooking was never a pleasure. It was a chore, one to be avoided whenever I could. When my children were young, I spent hours every day in the kitchen. Were my efforts appreciated? Not on your life. Every meal brought out a chorus of whiners. "Do we have to eat that?" "Not again." "Why did you make that awful stuff?" "Can't you give me something else to eat?" "I'd rather have chocolate ice cream." And "I'd rather starve than eat that yucky stuff." When the children weren't whining, they were holding their plates under the table and feeding their food to the dog. As soon as meal time was over, everyone disappeared and I was left alone in the kitchen to clean up the mess, put the dishes in the dishwasher, and put away the leftovers. And yes, there were piles of leftovers. When I served the leftovers the next

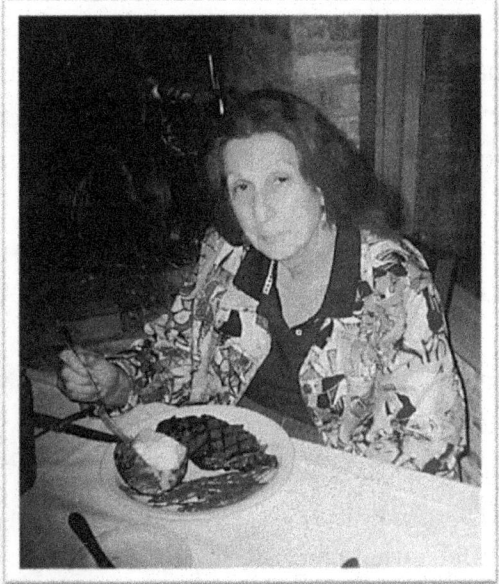

night, the whining was louder than it had been the night before. As you can guess, the only one who enjoyed my cooking, if you could call my lack of skill in the kitchen cooking, was our dog. Our little beagle-basset hound grew so fat on the leftovers that her stomach dragged across the ground and she waddled from side to side. The vet ordered me to put her on a diet.

When I was growing up, my father went to Davis Bakery very early every Sunday. He got there just as the bread was being taken out of the oven. Dad bought a couple of rye breads, Kaiser Rolls, and bagels. The smell of hot fresh rye bread was intoxicating. My mother loved the rye bread crust, and I favored its soft center. Each of us took the part of the loaf we liked best. By Sunday afternoon, the two of us had finished off a rye bread. Fortunately for her, no amount of food ever made her fat. I took after my father's side of the family. All I had to do was look at food and I put on weight.

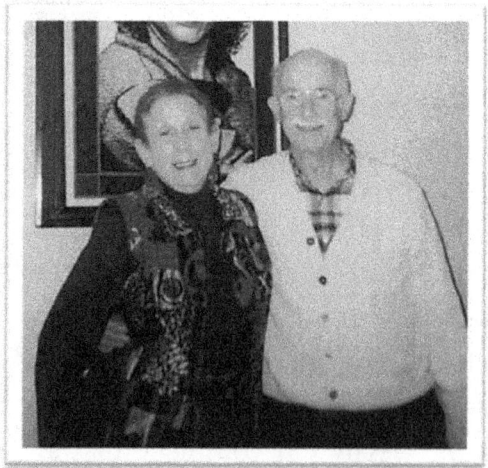

It was just my luck that my first husband's entire family was overweight. Bernard's family introduced me to fattening foods I had never had before – macaroni and cheese, salad dressing, pizza, stuffing, gelatin molds, fried chicken, *kugels, kreplach, kasha, schmaltz,* gravy on meat and potatoes, and pies and cakes with every meal. I have always had an aversion to fat. I do not like the taste and have always cut all the fat off my meat. Before I married, it was just thrown in the garbage. After I married, Bernard and his father would grab the fat off my plate and eat it. They told me I was missing the best part. All I could think of was, "yuck!"

In the 1960's I had yet to learn that circumstances and environment often determine people's eating habits. Bernard's father came to the United States from the Pale of Settlement in Russia. It was a walled-in area where the Czars forced the Jews to live. The inhabitants lived in wooden shacks, nearly froze to death in the winter, and had wolves at their doors scrounging for food. They were also subject to raiding parties who stole their food and possessions. On a good day they had barely enough food to sustain them. They ate whatever was available, including the fat on meat. It is also the area where *gribbenes* comes from. *Gribbenes* is made by cooking the chicken skin over a low heat to remove the fat. Onions are also browned in the chicken fat. Leftover from the rendering is *schmaltz;* a fat used in frying, baking, and mixing with other foods such as chopped liver, stuffing, and mashed potatoes. It is also spread across bread. Bernard's father grew up under these circumstances and became accustomed to them. He therefore passed these habits and preferences onto Bernard and his brother.

In the 1970's my dentist advised me to stop eating bread. Doctor Pleet said bread caused the rash of cavities I had. He said bread, especially white bread, sticks to the teeth and is difficult to remove. He also said he wished all his patients would give up eating bread. But we are a bread nation. Look at all the McDonalds, Burger Kings, Hardee's, Subways, Steak & Shakes, KFCs, Dairy Queens, Taco Bells and other fast food restaurant chains. Supermarket deli counters make sandwiches too. Sandwiches are the mainstay of their menus. And numerous sandwich selections fill sit-down restaurant menus too. Let's face it. It is easier to grab a sandwich and eat it on the run than it is to eat a meal that requires the use of a knife and fork. It is also quicker and more profitable for restaurants to slap together a sandwich than to take the time to cook food. Did I give up eating bread after my dentist told me to? No. Since I never really cared for white bread, I brought rye, challah, pumpernickel or onion bagels instead.

I became so fat that I gave up taking baths and opted for showers instead. It was too big a struggle for me to force my bulging stomach and hips out of the tub. In the shower, I gave up washing my feet because I couldn't bend over far enough to reach them. For two years the only one who appreciated my stinky feet was my dog. She cuddled up to my toes, licked them, and smiled like she was in heaven. Her slobber made them wet, sticky, and made me feel like I was trudging through marshland.

Like so many women who want to hide their expanding bodies, I spent years wearing navy, hunter green, gray, and black clothes. I wore clothes made from fabric with lots of stretch because natural fibers like cotton, wool, silk, and rayon did not have enough give in the areas where I needed it most. I also avoided wearing belts because I no longer had a waistline I wanted to show off. I was so uncomfortable that I also took to wearing muumuus and long dresses without waistlines around the house.

In the mid 1970's I took a course at Stretch n Sew® and began making clothes for our family. Synthetic fibers were cheap and easy to work with. I even made bathing suits for everyone but me. I wasn't going to embarrass myself by showing off my less than perfect body in public. Slacks, skirts, dresses, blouses, sweaters, and jackets were fine, but no one was ever going to get me into a bathing suit, not even one I could have made to cover up the areas I never wanted anyone to see. One day I looked in the mirror and noticed that the stretchy fibers clung to my body revealing every bulge, so I went to all my favorite shopping haunts and tried on natural fiber clothes in one size bigger than I normally wore. When I looked in the mirror I saw that I actually looked smaller because non-clingy clothes did not reveal the areas I wanted to hide the most. The artist in me also quickly discovered that I could distract people from staring at my large body if I wore big bold necklaces and huge dangling earrings. Best of all, jewelry was all one size; I never had to give up the pieces I liked when my girth increased. I must have been pretty good at hiding how huge I was because no one

ever guessed how many scales had broken under my weight. Today I
wear bright colors and prints. I am proud of my size and want everyone
to know it.

My weight loss
surprised me in another
area. All of my shoes and
boots became too big.
They fell off my feet. What
I didn't realize was that
when one is as heavy as I
was, your weight puts
extra pressure on your feet
which makes your feet
bigger, so you need bigger
shoes.

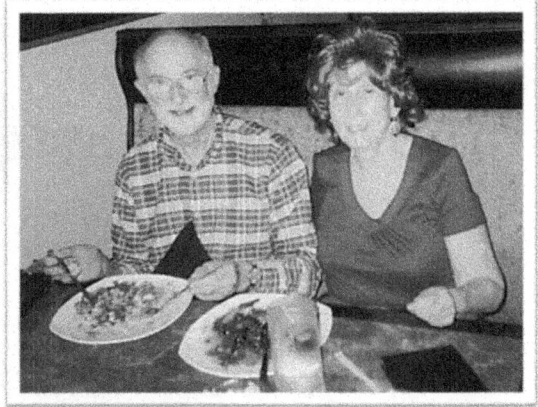

In the mid 1970's I met Carole, a mother on welfare. We became
the best of friends. Carole told me she ate bread every time she had a
migraine. I thought, "Yeah, right. Bread is going to cure my headache
when all the prescription drugs I took wouldn't." I assumed she ate the
bread because she could not afford to go to a doctor and get a
prescription. But as it turned out, she had the cure for my migraines.
On the rare occasion that I have a migraine, I eat two slices of bread
with butter in addition to taking the drug my doctor prescribed. I eat
rye, pumpernickel, sourdough, or challah, but not white bread. I don't
advise this cure for everyone, but it does work for me.

In the mid 1980's, John Malloy, the *Dress for Success* guru,
advised women to purchase their shirts and sweaters in the men's
department because similar clothing was more expensive in women's
departments. I bought large size shirts, sweaters, and quilted vests in
the men's departments not to save money but because they fit my
rotund figure better and were more comfortable and less constricting
than form-fitting women's apparel. In *Thursday's Child*, a collection
of forty-three short stories based on my life, the "Seventy-Five Cent

Coat" story relates how I came to purchase a royal blue Eddie Bauer Gore-Tex ® coat at a garage sale. See cover photos. I wore the coat for several years. After I went on my *Fat to Fabulous* restaurant lovers' diet, the coat hung on me. It looked like I was wearing a shapeless sleeping bag. Now my husband wears the coat and the men's shirts, sweaters, and quilted vests which also became too big on me.

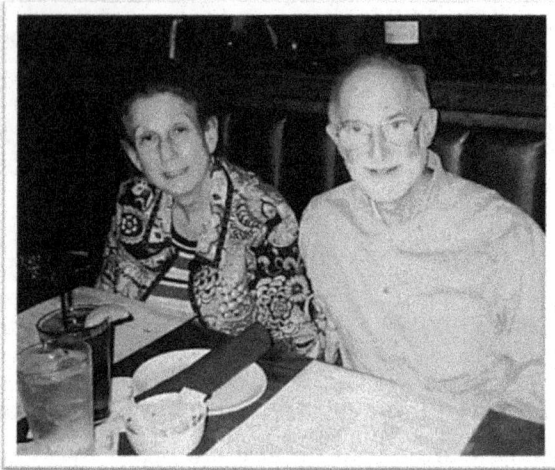

Sugar is put into processed foods to increase their shelf life and make them taste better. The American Heart Association and the U.S. Department of Agriculture recommend that we consume no more than six teaspoons of sugar per day, but how many people are going to spend their day looking at labels on fruit juice and soda bottles and cans and packages of processed meats and vegetables, yogurt and ice cream cartons, and cereal, cake, and cookie mix boxes? If you did, you'd spend all day in the supermarket doing nothing but reading labels. I don't know about you, but I don't have the time or the patience for that. For me, the best solution to the sugar problem is to avoid as many processed foods as possible and eat foods that are prepared fresh.

Even during World War II when there was strict rationing and women could only purchase a limited amount of sugar at the grocery store, sugar was used in abundant quantity in processed foods. To supplement his army pay, my father worked in one of California's fruit canneries. He said that after the cherries were washed, pitted, and thrown into the huge cooking vats, men stood over the vats throwing handfuls of sugar into the batch. "We never knew how much went into each batch because we never measured it," he said.

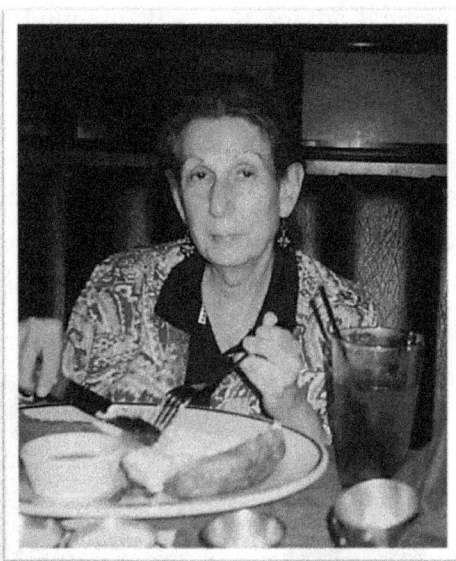

I read an article about a dentist who wanted to trace the origin of cavities. To do this, he went to art museums and studied Old Masters paintings. In Pieter Brueghel's paintings he found toothless Flemish people. Because sugar was not grown in Europe, he started studying shipping charts. He learned that in the 1500's merchants began importing sugar into Europe. In Brueghel's paintings he also discovered that after people began eating sugar they also became plump.

When we lived in Fort Worth, Texas in the 1980s, Doctor David Winter was a frequent guest on the evening news. Doctor Winter pointed out the high sugar content in pies, cakes, ice cream, cookies, snack foods, and sodas and advised dieters to restrict their sugar intake. These are the obvious sources. Either he never mentioned it or I missed it, but I never heard him talk about the less obvious sources of sugar. _Your medicine._ While doing research for the second edition of _From Fat to Fabulous: Another Diet Guide for Restaurant Lovers,_ I read books on diet and nutrition, calorie and carbohydrate counters, and books on pills and vitamin supplements. I could not find any mention of sugar contained in drugs in any of those sources. Actress Julie Andrews portrayed a fictional character in the movie "Mary Poppins". When she sang about a spoonful of sugar helping the medicine go down, she was telling it like it is. What I've said is _not_ intended as medical advice nor is it intended to make you give up the medicine you are taking. It is strictly to inform you that sugar is found in some of the most unlikely places.

In 1976 after my marriage to my first husband Bernard was annulled by the religious court, I became the sole support of two minor children and a dog. It was also the year that the bottom fell out of the home crafts market. I had been designing latchhook rug kits for Rapco and other crafts companies, and now I was out of a job. I found employment at Montgomery Wards selling, repairing, and teaching women how to use sewing machines. The hours were long. I did not earn enough to pay the mortgage, put food on the table, pay for babysitters, or provide all the things my two school-age children needed. When J.C. Penny offered me more money, I switched companies. Unfortunately the so-called higher pay turned out to be nothing more than a way to lure me away from Wards. I was repeatedly taken out of the sewing machine department to replace the men in major appliances when they went to lunch or dinner. The department manager gave my commissions to the men for every washer, dryer, refrigerator, or television set I sold. So not only did I lose commissions on the major appliances I sold but I also lost sales from the sewing machine department because I was absent from the department so often.

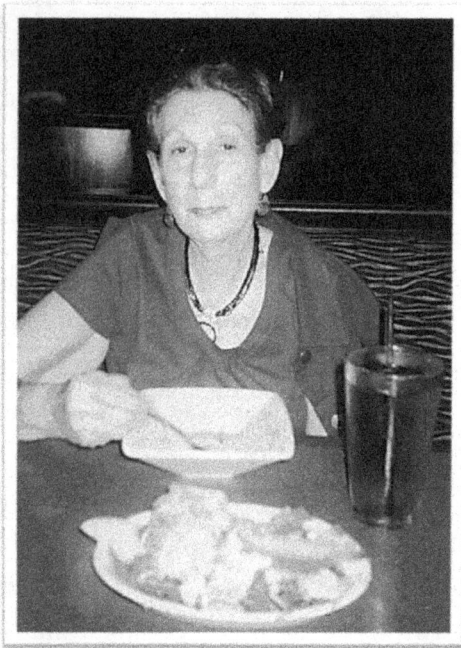

I also had a problem at home. My daughter repeatedly told me the babysitters I hired were not doing their job. They often showed up late, left the children standing outside the house waiting for them, did not give them dinner, and spent hours gabbing on the phone with their boyfriends. My solution to the problem was to give the house key to my daughter and leave dinner in the refrigerator for her and her brother. In spite of the fact that my daughter was a very responsible child, the police patrolling the area wanted an adult with them at all times. They were especially concerned about them being alone during the nights I had to work late and did not get home until 10:00pm.

1976 was also the year a new federal law demanded that manufacturers give women equal employment opportunities. Hoping to cure my financial problem and my situation at home at the same time, I contacted an employment agency. They sent me to Barre-National, a company in Baltimore, Maryland that manufactured Revco Drugs' generic drugs. In spite of the fact that my employment application listed me as an artist, Barre-National hired me to work in the weighing room, a job formerly reserved only for men.

When my weighing room partner, a tiny Asian woman, and I had to drag 600-pound barrels of chemicals from the storage room to the weighing room, I understood why men were preferred for the job

There was a heavy book in the weighing room which contained the formula for every drug manufactured in the United States. My partner, a chemist with a PhD, referred to the book as the "drug cookbook". Like a cookbook, it listed all the ingredients and the amounts needed to manufacture each drug. After measuring all the chemicals used in a specific drug, we ripped open huge bags of sugar and

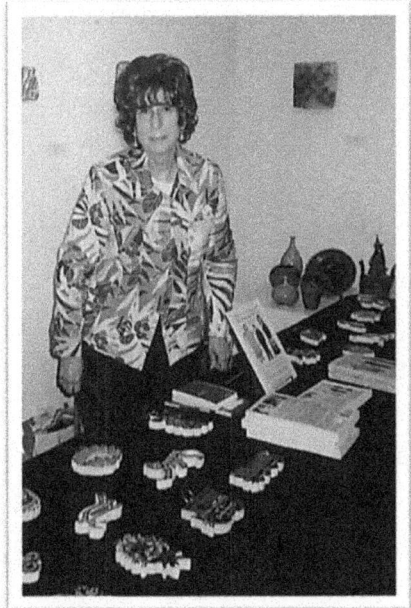

placed them in a separate container. The sugar and coloring added to it became the drug's outside coating. When I asked my partner why we needed the sugar, she said, "Because the drugs are so bitter people wouldn't be able to get them down." Back in 1976 I didn't think about what my weighing room partner said, but I do now. With all the medications I now take for my numerous health problems, I have to limit the sugars in what I eat in order to take weight off and keep it off.

The mid 1980's ushered in the era of the "big beautiful woman". Women's lib and the talk shows – Oprah, Sally, Morrie, Jessie, Phil Donohue, Montel and others – all venerated the "big beautiful woman". As an artist I was accustomed to seeing paintings depicting Rubenesque figures. Until the roaring 1920's ushered in the slim boyish figure, for centuries large women had set the standard for beauty. It was proof that a man could support his family. When every diet I tried failed, I bought into the "big is beautiful" concept. I decided if anyone did not like me the way I looked, they were not worth knowing. What I failed to see was while I was making excuses for my size, I was ruining my health. My doctors were no help at all. They said, "I'd rather see you overweight than see you taking off the weight and then putting it back on again. Yo-yo dieting is worse for your health." So they too handed me an excuse to stay fat. No talk show or doctor ever even suggested what the future consequences would be if I didn't lose the weight and keep it off. And believe me, there were consequences. Years later I became so heavy my knees gave out and I was not able to walk. They

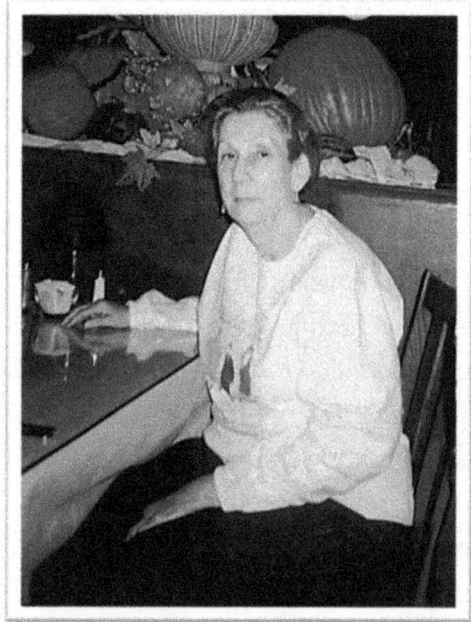

say a picture is worth a thousand words. If one of my well-meaning health care professionals had ever taken the time to show me pictures of the dire consequences I would face in the future because of my weight, I might have listened.

My restaurant lovers' diet is a godsend because I hate to cook. In the past, five minutes after I'd spent all day in the kitchen preparing and cooking a meal, my husband, the kids, and the dog the kids fed the food they didn't want to devoured it. It was followed by hours of cleanup without any help. Then I had to do it all over again the next day. Today I eat in restaurants or microwave my leftovers at home. It is *all pleasure* and *no work*.

Today, whenever there is a storm, the first thing I do is check the freezer to make sure my restaurant leftovers are still frozen. The second thing I do is check to see that the microwave is still functioning.

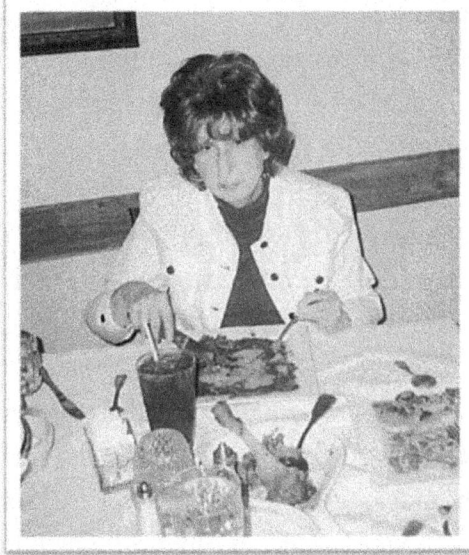

It has been four years since I last set foot in my kitchen to cook a meal. My daily prayer is - God willing, I will never have to cook another meal.

As the result of having a very smart Labrador retriever, I have had to make changes in my kitchen. My dog loves to play with the Corning Ware ® pots and pans I use to microwave my leftovers in. Kaya - her Native American name means wise child - lives up to her name. She discovered if she puts her mouth over the round knobs on our cupboard doors and backs up, she can open the bottom cupboards. Using her mouth and paws, she pulled and shoved my pots and pans out of the cupboards and dumped them on the kitchen floor. *POW! Bang! Crash!* Because we have ceramic tile floors in the kitchen, I was afraid she would break the pots and pans and get hurt on the sharp glass edges. So I now store my Revere Ware ® on the bottom shelves and the Corning Ware ® on

the top cupboard shelves. If not for Kaya dragging them out of the cupboard, my copper bottomed cookware would have never seen the light of day.

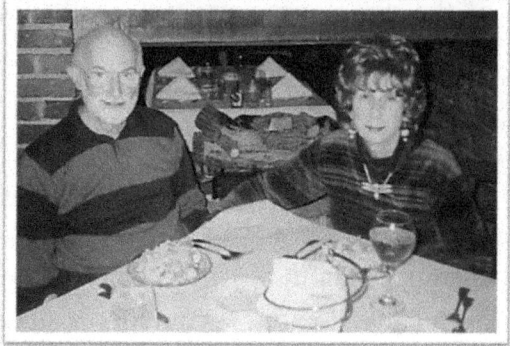

I have included the following story because *no* diet, including mine, will work if you cheat.

One evening my husband and I went out to dinner with a friend who had spent the last five years trying to lose weight. Mel had numerous health problems and his doctor had ordered him to lose a minimum of one hundred pounds. He was interested in my diet because he had joined one weight loss group after another, lost weight, and gained it right back.

Mel began dinner by ordering a Riesling wine. Shortly after the wine arrived, the waiter put a basket of Italian bread on the table. Mel tore off a section of the bread from the loaf, noticed the bottle of olive oil on the table, and flagged the waiter down.

"I'd like some butter," he said.

The waiter rolled his dark brown eyes toward the ceiling and an I*s he crazy?* look spread across his rugged face. He shrugged his shoulders as if to ask *He wants butter in an Italian restaurant?*

"Mel, wouldn't olive oil be a better . . .?"

I never got a chance to finish telling him olive oil would be a healthier and more sliming choice. He turned his head and looked around the room impatiently seeking the waiter's return. Mel smiled when the waiter finally placed a heaping plate of pads of butter on the table. Mel lifted several pads of butter off the dish and spread them liberally across his bread.

"You're looking great, Elaine. I've got to get a copy of your diet and follow it," he said as he tore off a second chunk of bread and buttered it.

Mel ordered the steamed mussels appetizer. He ate half of it and had the waiter box up the rest to take home.

"I'm watching my diet very carefully," he said with great pride. He took another piece of bread out of the basket and buttered it.

When the waiter came around again, Mel ordered another glass of wine. A chopped salad containing crispy prosciutto, tomatoes, blue cheese, avocado and a house dressing followed the mussels. He ate half of the salad and had the waiter box up the rest to take home. Then he ate more bread with butter. His entrée was the Rustic Chicken & Shrimp Forno specialty pasta. It consisted of ziti, prosciutto, Asiago cheese, shrimp, grilled chicken, and a red pepper cream sauce. Again he ate half and had the waiter box up the rest. He also put several pieces of bread and butter in the box.

"I'm really watching how much I eat," he said as he took more bread and butter.

I wanted to say "Mel, if you really want to lose weight, you're going to have to give up eating all that bread and butter and those large orders of pasta," but he was trying so hard to impress me claiming he was doing everything possible to lose weight I was not able to get the words out. For dessert he had the chocolate Zuccotto cake and a dessert wine. The slice of cake was big enough to feed four people, but Mel ate the whole thing.

In the first edition of *From Fat to Fabulous: A Diet Guide for Restaurant Lovers* I related the story of Gail and her inability to lose weight. Because readers asked if Gail ever took off the weight, I have decided to update Gail's story.

Every time I saw Gail, she appeared to have gained more weight. Chairs sagged under her, she waddled when she walked, and she could no longer bend over and see her feet. Somehow it is easier for me to tell a woman she has to lose weight than it is to tell a man. So every

time I went out to lunch with Gail and our writers' critique group I told
her she had to give up all the bread she eats.

"Elaine, how did you really take it off?" Gail asked every time she
saw me.

"With my restaurant lovers' diet," I answered.

To this day, Gail constantly moans, "Damn doctors. They blame
everything on my weight. They claim all my health problems are due
to my weight. They're just making excuses because they can't cure
me."

She had had several major life-threatening illnesses. Her doctors
had attributed them directly to her weight and had told her she had to
lose a minimum of one hundred pounds. She had had the help of
doctors, dietitians, nutritionists, and health and diet clubs but had never
been able to keep it off.

"I lose one hundred pounds and gain it right back, then lose it
again and regain it. I can't seem to keep it off," Gail whined.

At a recent luncheon the new perky slim ponytailed waitress put
a basket of bread on the table. Gail grabbed the loaf of bread, tore it
apart, and began dipping the bread in an olive oil, butter, and parmesan
cheese mixture.

Gail noticed me watching her. She smiled sweetly and in a
condescending tone said, "You don't need any bread, Elaine. You're
on a diet."

The smell of fresh home-baked sourdough bread wafted through
the air. I could see the other members of our group wanted a piece too.

"You're right about me being on a diet. But how about leaving
some bread for someone else?" I asked her.

"Don't worry, the waitress will bring some more," Gail replied.

She waved a big hand through the air as if waving away a pesky
fly.

A tall dark-haired busboy with the face of an angel arrived at our
table with another basket of bread. He noticed a basket was already on
the table and turned on his heel to deliver the bread to another table.

"No! Leave it!" Gail yelled.

She raised a hand as if reaching for the basket.

As soon as the busboy set the basket on the table, Gail grabbed the second basket and placed it by her plate. Again she was the only one at our table who got any bread. She ordered a small salad topped with salami and bleu cheese dressing for lunch. When it arrived, she took a few bites of her salad, said she was too full to finish it, and asked the busboy to wrap it up to take home for supper. She also had him pack up the bread she had not finished plus one additional loaf.

"Gail, there's no way you're ever going to lose weight eating all that bread," I said.

"I love it," she replied. "I can't get sourdough bread like this at home."

When the waitress came to our table again, Gail batted her eyelashes coyly and laced her thick ring-covered fingers over her more than ample stomach.

"It's my birthday." Her heavily mascaraed eyelashes fluttered up and down. "Do I get a piece of cake?"

"Yes, Ma'am, you do," the waitress said and rushed off to the kitchen.

While Gail waited for the cake to arrive, she asked our group to share it with her. But when the slice of chocolate cake arrived, Gail's eyes bulged out of their sockets.

"Um, yummy," she said, and flagged down the waitress to ask for a take-home container.

When the container arrived, Gail put the entire piece of cake in it.

"It'll be my dessert tonight." Her eyes lit up like she was thinking of the heavenly experience she would have. Her rouged cheeks turned bright pink.

Again I left the restaurant trying to figure out how to help Gail help herself, but I knew it was a losing battle.

From time to time our group visits one of our local museums. A thin hostess with an auburn braid ending at her waistline wearing a floor-length black evening skirt, a short sleeve sequined blouse, and sandals seated us in the museum's posh dining room. A pudgy waiter in slacks and a long sleeve dress shirt came to our table to take our drink order. Before any of us could get a word out, Gail whipped out her Triple A card. She looked up at him expectantly and flashed him the card.

"I get a piece of cake because I'm a Triple A member, don't I?" she asked. She sounded excited and acted like she was anticipating every bite.

The waiter coughed. "Ah, yes, Ma'am you do. I'll bring the dessert tray around after lunch and you can make your selection then. Now, what'll you have to drink?" He nodded in my direction but I never got a chance to answer.

"I'll have the cake now," Gail announced. "And be sure there's plenty of bread on the table too."

The waiter rolled his eyes toward the ceiling, took our drink orders, and hurried over to the bar to fill them.

"Gail, how did you know that you'd get a free piece of cake with your Triple A card?" I asked.

She smiled a huge know-it-all smile, rocked backward in the chair, and laced her hands over her more than ample stomach.

"I looked it up online, checked out every restaurant who gives a free dessert to Triple A members."

Gail licked her lips when she saw the dessert tray.

"Um, yummy. I'll have the carrot cake with a big scoop of ice cream. And don't forget to put lots of bread on the table."

When our teas and coffees and the silver basket containing the bread and butter arrived, Gail grabbed the basket and tore off a huge chunk of bread. When she noticed everyone looking at her, she shoved what was left of the bread into the center of the table. That afternoon, Gail's entire meal consisted of bread, butter, carrot cake, ice cream, and tea.

In a last ditch effort to try to get Gail change her eating habits, I brought a *Wall Street Journal* article to our writers' critique group and read it. "Obesity is Linked to Cancer Deaths. The risk of dying can be as much as 62% higher for heaviest Americans. . . . A 5-foot-4-inch woman would be considered obese if she weighed more than 174 pounds . . . A 6-foot man would be classified as obese if he weighed more than 221 pounds." Did Gail change her eating habits? No! The next time we went out to lunch, she ate more bread than she had on previous trips.

Obese individuals eat and think differently from their thin contemporaries. The obese ones I have met think and talk about food nonstop. It doesn't matter whether it's a man or a woman. I have noticed almost everyone who has trouble losing weight eats large amounts of bread, pasta, potatoes, rice, and dessert. Taking home half a meal the way Gail and Mel did does not help. They are still eating the very things that caused them to gain weight in the first place. These are the foods that should be eaten only on reward nights. Wine may be good for your heart, but overindulging like Mel did only adds pounds. On reward nights I limit myself to one glass of wine. I never eat shrimp, avocado, prosciutto, or any other pork product.

During our vacation my husband and I ate several meals at a posh salad bar in the southwest. The variety of salads, salad toppings, and desserts seemed almost endless. Our table was directly across from the salad bar. It gave me an opportunity to observe other diners without them knowing I was observing them. Without exception the obese diners put bacon, ham, and croutons on their salads. They also piled crackers, bread sticks, rolls, and butter on their plates. When they had a choice between the beef vegetable soup, green chili chicken tortilla soup without tortilla strips, or the lobster bisque, they chose the lobster bisque. Flour or cornstarch is used to thicken lobster bisque. For dessert, they chose the puddings, gelatins, and canned fruits slathered with heavy whipped cream instead of the fresh strawberries, pineapple, and melons.

In 1961 I took an oil painting class at Kent State University. My instructor set up a still life in one room and gave us five minutes to walk around it and study it. Then he locked the door and we had to return to the painting room and paint what we saw. This course greatly enhanced my ability to notice things and later recall what I saw. My husband thinks I see and hear more than the average

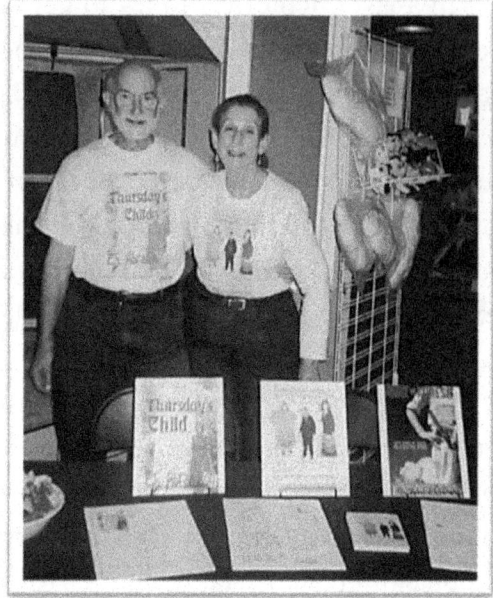

person does. I credit this course for that. When Stan began taking me to restaurants because I was in so much pain I could not stand in the kitchen long enough to prepare a meal, I watched what other diners ate. I quickly noticed a pattern. The heavier diners tended to order one type of food, and the thinner ones ordered another. I tried the foods the thinner diners ate but quickly became bored eating the same things over and over again. I had to strike a balance so I experimented until I found combinations that worked.

My restaurant lovers' diet has improved my health and given me a new lease on life. A *Java Journal* article listed foods to avoid if you want to have good health. Number one on the avoid list was all pork products, especially bacon, sausage, hot dogs, and pepperoni. These foods are also high on my avoid list. They contain huge amounts of fat, salt, food coloring, and nitrites which cause cancer. Number two on their list was shellfish because these ocean scavengers feed on fecal matter from other fish. Just reading about those foods was enough to make me glad they are not a part of my diet, but these are the foods that most overweight people seem to eat. They load up on hot dogs at ballparks, bacon and sausage in hotel and restaurant breakfasts, pepperoni on pizza and salads, and fried shrimp appetizers and meals. These foods provide little to no nutritional value. They harm the body and expand the waistline.

When I was a teenager, boys bragged about taking a bottle of cola and using it to clean rust off their cars. Recently the makers of sports drinks and sodas came under fire for putting brominated vegetable oil in their drinks. Change.org noted that this ingredient was patented as a flame retardant. The substance is banned in the European Union and Japan. The makers of these products also put sucrose acetate isobutyrate, a sugar substitute, in sports drinks and sodas to maintain the flavor and taste. Researchers have discovered people who drink low or no calorie drinks and beverages containing sugar substitutes tend to eat far more than people who do not drink them. People assume because these drinks contain few or no calories, they can eat more food. Friends have compared trying to stop drinking these beverages to being a drug addict going through detox. They said, "I get migraines, the shakes, and all sorts of weird out-of-body experiences." I don't know about anyone else, but it makes no sense to me to drink beverages that clean rust off cars, contain flame retardants, affect your health, and expand your waistline.

Diet books, weight loss groups, and nutritionists advise you to avoid eating at buffets. I love the infinite variety of foods at buffets, but I do pass up all fried foods, breads and pastas, potatoes, pork products, seafood, and foods coated with breading or flour. I eat a variety of salads, soups, steamed, grilled, and sautéed vegetables, and meats that are grilled, broiled, stewed, baked, or sautéed. I drink tea, coffee, or water. On the three reward nights a month that I treat myself to dessert, my husband and I share one dessert.

***

There are very few rules to my restaurant lovers' diet. When traveling I pass up the free breakfasts provided by the hotels because I do not eat hot or cold cereal, sausages, bacon, ham, toast, bagels, donuts, pastry, waffles, powdered eggs, or hash brown potatoes. AOL's travel writer claims "Hotels Serve Glorified Prison Food For Breakfast. I've never been to a prison, but I can't help but wonder if convicts get nicer breakfasts than what you find on the breakfast buffets at most American chain hotels these days." I only stay at hotels where I can have a refrigerator and microwave in my room so I can eat my previous night's restaurant leftovers.

Most restaurants will be happy to make changes when you request them. I do not eat any bread, bacon, ham, shellfish, fish or American cheese and do not drink soda. I rarely eat pasta, potatoes, rice, or dessert. The bread part can be a little tricky. Because menus often do not say that meat, vegetables, soups, or cheeses are coated with flour or bread crumbs, before ordering I always ask the waitperson if the food is prepared with them. When I order French onion soup, I ask the waitperson to tell the chef to leave out the bread and croutons. I order all salads without bacon and croutons. With veal, chicken, and eggplant I ask them not to use any breading or flour. I do not eat any bread or tortillas the waitperson puts on the table. I ask that all my food be prepared fresh. I do not want it frozen, prepackaged, or from boxes because food prepared in these manners often contain bread products and excessively large amounts of salt and sugar. They are the cheap fillers that made me fat. I trim every scrap of fat off my meat. That includes removing the skin from chicken and turkey. I never add salt or sugar to my food. I drink lots of regular or decaffeinated coffee or herbal tea with a low calorie sweetener or I drink water. My husband and I share appetizers, side salads, and soups. When we order a dessert on a reward night, we share them too. Both of us order our own main course.

Articles in the *Wall Street Journal* and *Town & Style* reported Ron Shaich, the co-chief executive officer of Panera Bread Company/St. Louis Bread Company/Paradise Bakery & Café, "is reducing his own consumption of baked goods and bagels". The article went on to say he had "lost 10 pounds after changing his diet and working out with a personal trainer." With my body by disaster, there is no way I would ever be able to do the high-impact exercises personal trainers recommend. My entire low-impact exercise regime consists of walking my dog and riding a stationary bicycle. I do not sacrifice any of the foods I love in order to lose weight. I do not know if Mr. Shaich ever read the first edition of *From Fat to Fabulous: A Diet Guide for Restaurant Lovers,* but I had given up eating bread long before I learned the co-chief executive officer of a large bakery chain had reduced his consumption of bakery products.

I order _all_ sandwiches open-faced. I have an aversion to fat and grease. I tried having restaurants leave off the bread or bun and use a paper towel to drain off the fat and grease, but that left the meat dry and tasteless. I like my meat juicy. I finally realized that since I do not eat the bread, I could use it to soak up the fat or grease, so I started having my sandwiches served open-faced.

Chocolate is the food of the gods. I am a chocoholic. No diet on this earth will ever make me give up my chocolate fix. My refrigerator is never without a supply of Lindt Excellence Intense Orange Dark Chocolate or Lindt Excellence 70% Cocoa Smooth Dark Chocolate bars. Every afternoon I eat two chocolate squares out of the ten squares or one fifth of a 3.5 ounce bar.

I have been a chocolate lover all my life. An *AARP Bulletin* said, "Choose chocolate. The sweet news about chocolate – that once-guilty pleasure – is that it has now become the darling of the heart-healthy diet." *The Atlantic* said, "Those who eat chocolate on a regular basis are thinner than those who don't, suggesting that the metabolic effects can more than offset additional calories." Wahoo! Fantastic! No one has ever had to tell me to eat chocolate. Now I can protect my heart and slim down at the same time. Living a long and healthy life has a lot to do with enjoying life. Chocolate and my restaurant lovers' diet make me very happy and help me do it.

All of the diets I have previously been on require the dieter to strictly follow the diet and never deviate from its rules in any way whatsoever. On my restaurant lovers' diet, three days per month and on special occasions I give myself a reward for losing weight and inches. For example, on my birthday I had a glass of Lambrusco and roasted potatoes with dinner and a large piece of decadent dark chocolate cake topped with whipped cream for dessert.

I eat until I feel full. Usually this amounts to approximately half of one entrée plus the appetizer, soup, and salad I share with my husband. The remainder of my entrée I take home. I discovered there is a big difference between drinking hot and cold beverages. I try to drink tea or coffee hot as often as possible because I feel full sooner and the feeling lasts longer.

When I began my diet I weighed myself once a week. Now I only weigh myself if I feel I might be slipping. I feel the true test of whether you are succeeding is if your clothes are getting too big on you. Before I started this diet, I spent my entire life buying clothes one size larger than I had bought previously. Now I have the joy of buying one size smaller. Every couple of months I donate my baggy old clothes to charity and purchase new ones. Best of all, it is the most wonderful feeling in the world to hear my family and friends tell me how great I look. My husband likes to go shopping with me. He enjoys seeing me model the clothes I intend to purchase. It gives him a chance to have his input about my wardrobe. Women who were total strangers have come up to me after I have shown my husband the outfits I intended to buy and have said they wished they could wear the same size clothes I now wear.

As my diet progressed I became more adventuresome. I wanted to try foods I had never eaten before, but this posed a problem. In many restaurants the waitstaff only knew what was printed on the menu. Most waitpersons will gladly go to the kitchen and ask the chef what are ingredients in the dish, but I found this to be time consuming, especially in crowded restaurants where the waitperson had several tables to serve. What usually happens is the waitperson takes orders from several tables, turns all of them in to the kitchen, and asks the chef your questions at the same time. I decided it was better to be an informed diner, so I purchased Baron's *Food Lover's Companion* and *Webster's New World Dictionary of Culinary Arts.* Both dictionaries give information about the ingredients in different dishes and methods of preparation. Before we try a new restaurant, my husband previews its menu online and prints it out. Then I look up any unfamiliar foods I want to try in my food dictionaries.

Dishes containing bread or wheat products are not always obvious. There is a Turkish restaurant my husband and I wanted to try. He printed off the menu and I saw tabbouleh listed under salads. Tabbouleh is a Middle Eastern dish made from Bulghur wheat, tomatoes, onions, parsley, mint, olive oil, and lemon juice. My food dictionaries listed wheat as the main ingredient in tabbouleh. So, for the salad I shared with my husband, I ordered a lettuce, tomato, green pepper, carrot, onion, olive oil, and lemon juice salad instead.

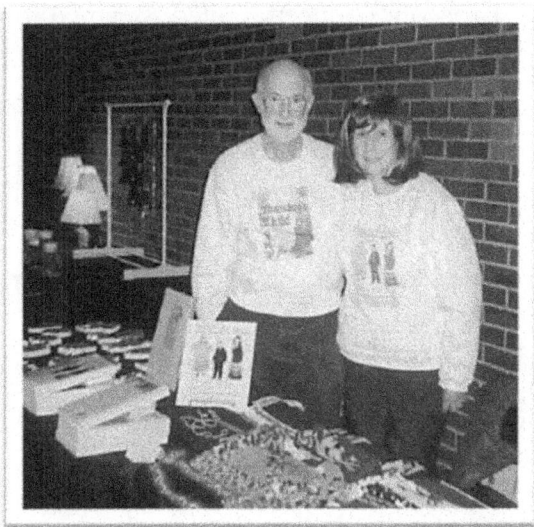

After the first edition of *From Fat to Fabulous: A Diet Guide for Restaurant Lovers* was released, several people told me they thought I did not eat any foods containing carbohydrates. Wrong! Aside from meat and cheese, just about every food contains some carbohydrates. You cannot eliminate them completely from your diet. I believe there are good carbohydrates and bad carbohydrates, both manmade and natural. Most of my carbohydrates are made by Mother Nature, not man. Below is a partial list of the carbohydrates I eat on a fairly regular basis. I did not list any of the manmade carbohydrates I eat on reward nights. Even though I am giving you carbohydrate statistics, like most people I do not pay attention to any statistics when I dine in a restaurant. I had to look up the carbohydrate count for each food in Prevention Magazine's *Nutrition Advisor* to find out what they were in order to tell you about them.

***

Almonds, dried, unblanched, unsalted – 5.8g per ounce.

Apples, fresh – 21.1g per 5 ounces. I eat them in salads.

Asparagus, steamed, broiled, boiled – 4.0g per half cup.

Blue cheese or Roquefort salad dressing, regular – 2.3g per 2 tablespoons.

Broccoli, chopped, boiled, steamed, broiled – 4.0g per half cup.

Cabbage, common, shredded, uncooked, boiled – 3.6g per half cup.

Cabbage, red, shredded, uncooked, boiled – 3.5g per half cup.

Carrots, raw – 7.3g per 2 ½ oz.

Cherries, sweet – 24.0g per cup without the pits. I eat about a quarter cup for dessert.

Chives, raw, chopped – 0.1g per tablespoon.

Chick-peas, canned – 27.1g per half cup. I sprinkle a few on top of my salad.

Cranberries – 6.0g per half cup. I eat them on salads.

Green peas, fresh – 12.5g per half cup boiled. I sprinkle a few on top of my salad.

Horseradish, prepared – 0.5 per teaspoon. I use it on steaks, ribs, and other meats.

Italian salad dressing, regular – 3.0g per 2 tablespoons.

Lettuce, iceberg, raw, shredded – 2.8g per cup.

Lettuce, Romaine, shredded, raw – 1.3g per cup.

Lindt Excellence Intense Orange Dark Chocolate bars – one serving is 4 squares or 40g. I eat two squares a day.

Mango – 17.6g per 3 ½ ounces. I eat them on Asian salads.

Mayonnaise – 0.4g per tablespoon.

Mushrooms, raw, boiled, cut in pieces – 4.0g per half cup.

Mustard, prepared, yellow – 1.0g per tablespoon.

Nuts, mixed, dry-roasted, unsalted – 7.2g per ounce.

Onions, chopped, boiled, raw, grilled – 6.9g per half cup.

Orange juice – 25.8g per 8 ounce glass.

Oranges – 15.4g per 4 ½ ounces. I eat them on salads.

Pecans, dry, unsalted, no sugar – 5.2g per ounce. I eat them on salads.

Peanuts, dry-roasted, unsalted – 6.0g per ounce.

Peppers, green or red bell, chopped, raw – 3.2g per half cup.

Pickles, sour – 0.8g per 1 ounce.

Pineapple, fresh – 19.2g per cup cut in cubes. I eat about half a cup for dessert.

Pine nuts, Pignolia, dried – 4.0g per ounce. I eat them on salads and mixed in with other foods.

Sesame seeds, dried, hulled – 0.8g per tablespoon. I eat them on salads, chicken, and steamed and grilled vegetables.

Spinach, boiled, raw – 3.4g per half cup.

Squash, Zucchini, raw, boiled, broiled – 3.5g per half cup.

Strawberries, fresh – 10.5g per cup. I eat strawberries with my breakfast.

Sunflower seeds, dries – 5.3g per ounce. I eat about a quarter of an ounce on salads.

Tea- 0.5g brewed per 6 ounce cup.

Tea, herbal – 0.4 per 6 ounce cup.

Tomato juice canned – 7.7g per 6 ounce glass. I usually prefer tomato juice over orange juice.

Tomatoes, raw – 5.7g per 4 ounces.

Water chestnuts, canned – 8.7g per half cup.

***

In _all_ restaurants, for breakfast I choose one entrée plus decaf coffee or tea with a low calorie sweetener.

In _all_ restaurants, for lunch or dinner I choose one appetizer, one soup, and one side salad to share with my husband. I order my own entrée and iced or hot tea with a low calorie sweetener. He drinks water or wine with dinner. When I ask the waitperson to leave off seafood or ham, at most restaurants they will ask if I want something in place of it. I order an extra salad or vegetable.

On reward days I choose one dessert and share it with my husband.

The restaurants mentioned in my restaurant lovers' guide are here because their owners or managers gave me copies of their menus and have been gracious enough to answer my questions. Their management and wait staff are a wonderful group of men and women. In order to be in this guide, the restaurant must serve its meals on plates and provide knives and forks. The necessity for these utensils will become more obvious as you view the selections my husband and I made from the menus the restaurants provided and read my comments. The only menu selections that appear in _From Fat to Fabulous: A Diet Guide for Restaurant Lover_ are the foods that my husband and I eat. We have eaten at all of the establishments listed in this guide. Their menus are arranged in alphabetical order.

I attend numerous art and craft shows and book signings each year. At various times I watch people walking up the aisles stopping at various booths. Seeing four and five hundred pound women struggling behind walkers to make it up the aisle made me realize at the rate I was putting on weight if I hadn't discovered my restaurant lovers' diet it wouldn't have been long before I would have become one of them. So now, every time I am in danger of not staying on my diet, I remember them and the horrible pain I had in my knees that necessitated my losing weight. I sympathize with their pain and struggles and know that for the sake of my health I can never return to being as heavy as I once was.

In some cases restaurants themselves make it difficult for diners to stick to their diets. I have repeatedly heard people who are taking the anticoagulant Coumadin (generic name Warfarin) complain the only vegetable option restaurants offer in place of potatoes, rice, or pasta is broccoli. *Dangerous Drug Interactions, The People's Pharmacy ® Guide* makes it clear that eating broccoli when one is on Coumadin is dangerous.

The restaurants leave dieters on Coumadin two options: eat the foods that add weight and inches to the waistline or tell the waitperson to leave these foods off their plate. In the interest of making diners healthier and happier, I would like to see restaurants offer green beans, steamed or grilled mixed vegetables, or dinner salads in place of the potatoes, rice, or pasta.

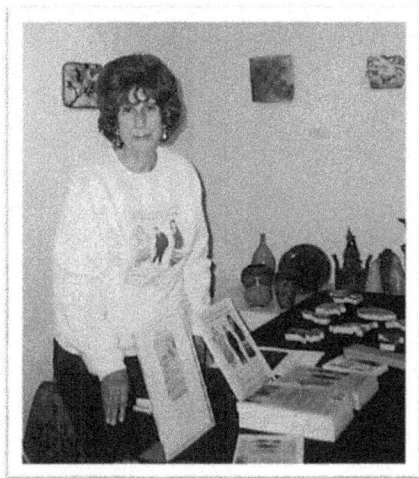

After the first edition of *From Fat to Fabulous: A Diet Guide for Restaurant Lovers* was published, I did a series of book signings. Women studied the three photographs of me on the cover. One shows the huge shapeless dress I wore 85 pounds ago. The second was taken after I lost the first 10 pounds. The third is how I look today. Their eyes popped out. They said, "Was that really you?" "Wow!" "What a way to go, sister." Many put their arms around me, hugged me, and said, "I'm so proud of you." Men pointed to the cover and said, "You really are fabulous." I hope you too will enjoy the fantastic high the compliments from people who have seen the results of my diet have brought me. It is the most wonderful feeling in the world to have people validate your success.

I hope you enjoy my restaurant diet as much as I do.

Happy eating,
Elaine

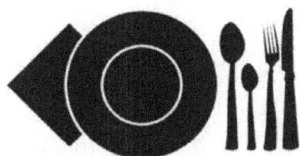

THE RESTAURANTS

BREAKFAST

<u>Blue Owl Restaurant & Bakery</u>

Kimmswick, MO

<u>Breakfast Quiche</u> – Served with fresh fruit cup

Side Orders

> Eggs

> Egg beaters

First Watch

Chain Restaurant

Omelets:

Served with either dressed greens or fresh, seasoned potatoes and an English muffin. Cholesterol/fat-free eggs or egg whites may be substituted at no additional charge. I order the fresh greens.

Killer Cajun® - Spicy Cajun all natural white-meat chicken breast with house roasted Crimini mushrooms, onions and Monterey Jack. Served with a side of Santa Fe sauce.

Greek Fetish® - Roasted red peppers, spinach, onions with feta and black olives.

C'est La Vie – House-roasted zucchini, onions and tomatoes with herbed goat cheese.

Veg'd Out™ - House-roasted Crimini mushrooms, zucchini, onions, tomatoes and broccoli with cheddar and Monterey Jack.

The Forager – House-roasted Crimini mushrooms and tomatoes with fresh herbs, mozzarella and Swiss.

Swiss Room - Ham, house-roasted Crimini mushrooms and onions with fresh herbs and Swiss. I ask the waitperson to ask the chef to substitute extra mushrooms for the ham.

First Watch® Eggs-clusives:

Caps, Etc.® - House-roasted Crimini mushrooms topped with melted cheddar and Monterey Jack. Served with two fresh eggs any style and an English muffin. I ask the waitperson to substitute extra cheddar for the English muffin.

Turkey Chive Crepegg® - A thin crepe layered with eggs, turkey, spinach, house-roasted onions and Monterey Jack.

Topped with diced tomatoes, chives and hollandaise. Served with an English muffin. I ask the waitperson to ask the chef to substitute extra tomatoes for the English muffin.

Noshville Delicatessen

Nashville, TN

Egg Dishes:

Served with choice of silver $ potato cakes, fresh fruit, oatmeal, sliced tomatoes, toast, or bagel. I order all my eggs with sliced tomatoes.

Egg Dishes:

> 2 Eggs Any Style
>
> Eggs and Onions

Omelets:

> Spinach & Cheese Omelet
>
> Vegetable Omelet
>
> Western Omelet – I ask the waitperson to ask the chef to leave out the ham.
>
> Create Your Own Omelet
>
> Spicy Chicken & Pepper Jack Cheese Omelet
>
> Tomato & Cheese Omelet

Check This Out!:

Potato Pancakes – I eat potato pancakes on a reward day.

Cheese Blintzes

Range Café

Albuquerque & Bernallio, NM

Breakfast:

Served until 3pm.

Range Favorites;

<u>N.Y. Steak & Eggs</u> – 7 oz. grilled N.Y. steak, two eggs cooked any style, sliced tomatoes, Range fries, and choice of bread. I ask the waitperson to ask the chef to substitute extra tomatoes for the Range fries.

Omelettes:

<u>Veggie</u> – Sun-dried tomato, avocado, red bell pepper, green onion, fresh tomato, fresh basil, white cheddar, cream cheese. I ask the waitperson to ask the chef to substitute extra tomato for the avocado and cheddar cheese for the cream cheese.

<u>I-25</u>- (it'll get you to Denver!) ham, bell pepper, onion, white cheddar cheese, topped with your choice of chili. I ask the waitperson to ask the chef to substitute extra bell pepper and onion for the ham.

<u>Tuscan</u> – Fresh spinach, artichoke hearts, sun-dried tomato, avocado, topped with pistachio pesto. I ask the waitperson to ask the chef to substitute onion for the avocado.

Weck's

Albuquerque, Santa Fe, Rio Rancho, and Los Lunas, NM

"Full Belly" Omelettes:

Four eggs served with fresh hash browns, toast or tortilla. On all Omelettes I ask the waitperson to ask the chef to substitute extra vegetables for the hash browns and the toast/tortillas.

Farmers Market – Sautéed mushrooms, onions, bell peppers, sprouts, diced tomatoes, and guacamole, sour cream, and cheddar and Jack cheeses, with your choice of red and/or green chili. I ask the waitperson to ask the chef to substitute extra cheddar for the guacamole.

The Abney – Diced bacon, fresh bell peppers, diced tomatoes, and guacamole, cheddar and Jack cheeses, with your choice of red and/or green chili. I ask the waitperson to ask the chef to substitute extra bell peppers and tomatoes for the bacon and the guacamole.

Healthier Alternative – Fresh onions, mushrooms, bell peppers, sprouts, and diced tomatoes folded into cholesterol-free egg substitute, eggs or egg whites topped with fresh diced green chili and served with sliced tomatoes and dry toast. (Veggies are served uncooked.) I order the eggs.

South of Denver Omelette – Diced ham, sautéed bell peppers and onions with cheddar and Jack cheeses and your choice of red and/or green chili. I ask the waitperson to ask the chef to substitute diced tomatoes for the diced ham.

Build Your Own Omelette – Start with a fluffy four egg Omelette and a blend of cheddar and Jack cheeses with your choice of red and/or green chili. Add your favorite ingredients (additional charge). Bell pepper, sautéed mushrooms, chopped green chili, sautéed onions, diced tomatoes, sprouts or sour cream.

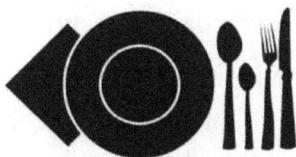

THE RESTAURANTS

LUNCH/DINNER

Artichoke Café

Albuquerque, New Mexico

Lunch:
Starters:

Steamed Artichoke – Clarified butter, raspberry vinaigrette, lemon-caper aioli.

Roasted Garlic – Montrachet goat cheese, roasted red peppers, oven-roasted olives, grilled baguette.

Soup Du Jour – Chef's daily selection.

Garden Salad – Mixed greens, tomato, red onion, cucumber, choice of ranch, Dijon vinaigrette, or blue cheese. I ask the waitperson to ask the chef to substitute extra tomato for the cucumber.

Entrées: - Add a garden salad or soup to any entrée.

Apple & Blue Cheese Salad – Mixed greens, endive, red grapes, candied marcona almonds, apple cider vinaigrette. I ask the waitperson to ask the chef to substitute extra mixed greens for the grapes.

Grilled Organic Chicken Salad – Baby spinach, mixed greens, marinated cucumber, carrot, toasted cashews, curry aioli. I ask the waitperson to ask the chef to substitute extra mixed greens for the marinated cucumber.

Grilled Greek Lamb Salad – Grilled eggplant, beefsteak tomato, caper berries, cucumber, garbanzo beans, feta, preserved lemon vinaigrette. I ask the waitperson to ask the chef to substitute extra tomato for the cucumber.

Grilled Sliced Steak – Angel hair pasta, pine nuts, basil, asparagus, roasted red pepper, cherry tomatoes, mixed greens, balsamic vinaigrette, and parmesan. I eat this dish on a reward day.

Gourmet Burger – Poppy seed bun, choice of two toppings: cheddar, Swiss, green Chile, artichoke hearts, mushrooms, roasted red peppers, herb French fries. I ask the waitperson to ask the chef to substitute an extra vegetable for the French fries.

Steak Frites – 6 oz. flat iron steak, herb French fries, maître d'hôtel butter, brandy demi-glace. I ask the waitperson to ask the chef to substitute a vegetable for the French fries.

Crepe of the Day – Chef's daily creation; served with fresh vegetables and fresh fruit.

Add grilled chicken for an additional charge.

Dinner:
Appetizers:

Steamed Artichoke – Clarified butter, raspberry vinaigrette, lemon-caper aioli.

Roasted Garlic – Montrachet goat cheese, roasted red peppers, oven-roasted olives, grilled baguette.

Cheese Plate – Assorted cheeses with garnishes.

Salads & Soups:

Apple & Blue Cheese Salad – Mixed greens, endive, red grapes, candied marcona almonds, apple cider vinaigrette. I ask the waitperson to ask the chef to substitute extra mixed greens for the grapes.

French Onion Soup Gratinee – Crostini and gruyere. I ask the waitperson to ask the chef to prepare my onion soup without the crostini.

Soup Du Jour – Chef's daily selection.

Entrées:

Grilled Dry-Aged Twelve Once Ribeye – Horseradish-cheddar mashed potatoes, apple cider vinegar braised greens, balsamic steak sauce. I eat this dish on a reward night.

Pan-Roasted New Zealand Lamb Rack – Quinoa pilaf, goat cheese, grilled escarole, mint, and lamb jus. I ask the waitperson to ask the chef to leave the mint off. I eat this dish on a reward night.

Veal Scaloppini Carbonara – Pancetta, English peas, tomato confit, fettuccini, cream, parmesan cheese. I ask the waitperson to ask the chef to substitute extra peas for the pancetta. I eat this dish on a reward night.

Pan-Roasted Free Range Chicken Breast – Goat cheese-mushroom stuffing, olive oil-parmesan polenta, broccolini, marsala pan sauce.

Steak Frites – 6 0z. grilled flat iron steak, house fries, maître d'hôtel butter, and brandy demi-glace. I ask the waitperson to ask the chef to substitute a vegetable for the house fries.

Sides:

Haricot Verts

Grilled Vegetables

Grilled asparagus

Big Vern's Steakhouse

Shamrock, TX

Steaks:

Served with one side, garden fresh salad or homemade vegetable beef soup, and fresh hot bread with whipped butter.

    16 oz. Ribeye

    2 oz. Ribeye

    10 oz. New York Strip

    8 oz. Filet Mignon

    8 oz. Ranch Sirloin

Entrées:

Served with hot bread, whipped butter, and garden fresh salad or homemade vegetable beef soup.

Chopped Sirloin – Served with caramelized mushrooms and onions, and choice of potato. I order the salad and ask the waitperson to ask the chef to substitute the soup for the potato.

Grilled Chicken Breast – Tender grilled chicken breast, topped with pepper Jack cheese, caramelized peppers and onions served over a bed of rice pilaf and a choice of one side. I order the salad and ask the waitperson to ask the chef to substitute the soup for the rice pilaf.

Grilled Lemon Butter Chicken Breast – Tender chicken breast grilled with lemon butter sauce and topped with grilled lemons and a choice of one side.

Side Dishes:

Caramelized Mushrooms and Onions

Steamed Vegetables

 Grilled Vegetables

Salads:

House Salad – Spring mixed baby greens and fresh green leaf lettuce topped with tomatoes, cucumbers and onions. I ask the waitperson to ask the chef to substitute extra tomatoes for the cucumbers.

Grilled Chicken Salad – Spring mixed baby greens and fresh green leaf lettuce topped with grilled chicken, sliced tomatoes, cucumbers, onions, real bacon crumbles and your choice of dressing. I ask the waitperson to ask the chef to substitute extra tomatoes and green leaf lettuce for the cucumbers and the bacon.

Sandwiches:

Grilled Chicken Sandwich – Grilled chicken breast served on a hamburger bun along with mayonnaise, tomatoes, and lettuce and chips or French fries. I ask the waitperson to ask the chef to substitute a vegetable for the chips or fries.

Hamburger Platter – Fresh grilled burger made to order along with chips or homemade fries. Cheese is an additional charge. I ask the waitperson to ask the chef to substitute a vegetable for the chips or fries.

BBQ Beef Sandwich – Served with onions and pickles along with your choice of fries or chips. I ask the waitperson to ask the chef to substitute a vegetable for the chips or fries.

Soup:

Homemade Vegetable Beef Soup

Desserts:

Bread Pudding

Bowl of Ice Cream

Black Angus Steakhouse

Chain Restaurant

Steakhouse Starters:

Teriyaki Steak Lettuce Cups – Skewers of steak, onions, and baby portabella mushrooms marinated in sesame-teriyaki. Served with crisp lettuce cups and our signature pineapple pico de gallo.

Fire-Grilled Fresh Artichoke – Served with tangy lemon aioli and basil pesto mayo for dipping.

Salads:

Filet Mignon Cobb Salad – Crisp greens, tossed with our house vinaigrette and topped with flame-grilled filet mignon, fresh avocado, tomato, Applewood-smoked bacon and bleu cheese crumbles. I ask the waitperson to ask the chef to substitute extra crisp greens and tomato for the avocado and the smoked bacon.

Chicken Cobb Salad – Crisp greens, tossed with our house vinaigrette and topped with grilled chicken, fresh avocado, tomato, Applewood-smoked bacon and bleu cheese crumbles. I ask the waitperson to ask the chef to substitute extra crisp greens and tomato for the avocado and the smoked bacon.

Burger and Sandwiches:

Partnered with coleslaw.

Steakhouse Bacon Cheeseburger – A half-pound of ground beef stacked with cheddar cheese, smoky bacon and onion rings. I ask the waitperson to ask the chef to substitute lettuce and tomato for the bacon and onion rings.

Chicken, Avocado & Bacon Sandwich – A grilled chicken breast topped with Monterey Jack cheese, fresh avocado, ripe tomato, Applewood-smoked bacon and a creamy parmesan sauce. I ask the waitperson to ask the chef to substitute extra cheese and tomato for the bacon and avocado.

Filet Mignon Sandwich – Sliced filet mignon topped with sautéed onions and red bell peppers, cheddar cheese and chipotle mayo,

Fixin's:

Our entrées come with the fixin's you crave. Served with warm, sweet molasses bread and partnered with ANY TWO of our 16 craveable sidekicks.

Garden Salad

Caesar Salad

Wedge Salad

Coleslaw

Steak Soup

Steamed Broccoli with shaved parmesan.

Sidekicks:

For an additional charge you can add them to your entrée.

Sautéed Sweet Onions.

Sautéed Fresh Baby Portabella Mushrooms

A combination of onions and mushrooms.

Prime Rib:

Seasoned, seared and slow roasted. Served with your choice of fresh or creamy horseradish sauce, and au jus.

Black Angus Fire-Grilled Steaks:

We proudly serve Black Angus beef, aged a minimum of 21 days.

Top Sirloin, Center-Cut – 8 oz. or 11 oz.

Sesame-Teriyaki Top Sirloin – Glazed with our house-made sesame-teriyaki sauce with fresh garlic, sesame and ginger.

Full-Flavored Rib Eye Steak – 12 oz. or 16 oz.

Bacon & Bleu Butter Rib Eye – Our full-flavored rib eye topped with bacon & bleu cheese butter. 12 oz. or 16 oz. I ask the waitperson to ask the chef to leave off the bacon.

New York Strip, Center-Cut – 12 oz. or 14 oz.

Filet Mignon, Center-Cut – 6 oz. or 8 oz.

Mushroom & Bleu Filet Mignon – Topped with sautéed baby portabella mushrooms and melted bleu cheese crumbles. 6 oz. or 8 oz.

Truffled Flat Iron – A flavorful 8 oz. flat iron steak topped with a decadent black truffle butter and sautéed baby portabella mushrooms.

More from the Grill:

Fire-Grilled Chicken – Two juicy chicken breasts lightly marinated with lemon, Rosemary, garlic and thyme.

Sesame-Teriyaki Chicken Breast – Two juicy chicken breasts glazed with our house-made sesame-teriyaki sauce with fresh garlic, sesame and ginger.

Campfire Feast for Two:

Appetizer – Your choice of any Steakhouse Starter to share.

Entrées - Choose any two entrées listed. Each entrée is served with any two craveable Sidekicks.

Top Sirloin – 8 oz.

New York – 12 oz.

Rib Eye – 12 oz.

Prime Rib – 8 oz.

Filet Mignon – 6 oz.

Desserts – Round out your feast with any one of our decadent desserts.

Blueberry Hill

Restaurant & Music Club
St. Louis, MO

Appetizers & Side Orders:

Our canola/corn frying oil contains zero trans fats. For dipping, add nacho cheese, ranch or house dressing.

Cheddar Cheese Balls

Veggie Sticks (with ranch dressing)

Zucchini Sticks

Fresh Fruit

Coleslaw

Chicken Breast

Cheese Plate

Salads:

Dressings -

House (Creamy Italian)

Balsamic Vinaigrette

Honey-Dijon

Ranch

Bleu Cheese

Chef Salad – Our house salad with turkey, ham, salami, provel cheese and artichoke hearts. Garnished with black olives, pepperoncini and tomato. I ask the waitperson to ask the chef to substitute extra turkey for the ham.

House Salad – Assorted lettuces, carrots, cucumbers, radicchio, radishes and red onions. Garnished with tomato. I ask the waitperson to ask the chef to substitute extra lettuce and tomato for the cucumbers and radicchio.

Garden Salad – Our house salad with celery, green peppers and provel cheese. Garnished with a wedge of hardboiled egg and tomato. I ask the waitperson to ask the chef to substitute extra lettuce and tomato for the cucumbers and radicchio.

Garden Salad Plus – Served with a charbroiled boneless chicken breast. I ask the waitperson to ask the chef to substitute extra lettuce and tomato for the cucumbers and radicchio.

Soup & Salad – Cup of soup with a large house salad, with chili, or French onion soup.

Soups:

Made fresh in our kitchen.

French Onion – Served with French bread and butter. I ask the waitperson to ask the chef to prepare my soup without any croutons.

Chili – Award-winning chili (spicy) garnished with cheddar cheese.

Gazpacho – Chilled Spanish soup of minced tomatoes, green peppers and onions (a bit spicy). Served with home style croutons. I ask the waitperson to ask the chef to leave off the croutons.

Soup du Jour – Please ask about our selection.

Hamburgers:

Bleu, Cheddar (soft spread), Swiss, Provel, Pepper or Goat Cheese are an extra charge.

Sautéed mushrooms or grilled onions are also an extra charge.

Hickory Burger – 5 oz. or 7 oz. all-natural hickory-seasoned hamburger with hickory sauce.

Famous 7 oz. Hamburger – Award-winning hamburger served on fresh sesame seed bun – 100% pure ground chuck. Also available in 5.75 oz. version.

Wagyu Sliders – Three 2 oz. Australian Wagyu beef sliders with American cheese. Served with chips. I ask the waitperson to ask the chef to substitute Swiss cheese for the American cheese and to substitute a vegetable for the chips.

Turkey Burger – 5 oz. ground turkey patty seasoned with black pepper and garlic.

Sandwiches:

Choice of bread or Kaiser rolls. Served with a pickle wedge and potato chips. Bleu, Cheddar (soft spread), Swiss, Provel, Pepper or Goat cheese are an extra charge.

Special Sandwich – Cold roast beef, ham and salami served on a large Kaiser roll with Swiss and provel cheeses, 1000 Island, lettuce, tomatoes and red onions. I ask the waitperson to ask the chef to substitute extra roast beef for the ham and to substitute Honey-Dijon for the 1000 Island dressing.

Reuben – Quite possibly the best in St. Louis. Corned beef on grilled marble rye with Swiss cheese, sauerkraut and 1000 Island dressing. I ask the waitperson to ask the chef to substitute mustard for the 1000 Island dressing.

French Dip – Hearty portion of roast beef on French bread, au jus.

Steak Sandwich – Seasoned sliced sirloin with choice of cheese on a hoagie roll. Grilled green peppers and onions are an additional charge.

Chicken – Broiled or Jerk (seasoned) chicken breast filet.

Speedwalker – Cup of Gazpacho with turkey sandwich on choice of bread. Fresh fruit garnish. No chips. No pickle. No substitutions. No temptation.

Blue Owl Restaurant & Bakery

Kimmswick, MO

Salads:

Fresh Tossed Salad - Crisp iceberg and romaine lettuce mixed with a variety of garden vegetables. Served with your choice of dressing and homemade croutons. I ask the waitperson to ask the chef to substitute extra vegetables for the croutons.

Tossed Strawberry Salad – Crisp iceberg and romaine lettuce tossed with fresh sliced strawberries, cheddar and Monterey Jack cheese and our delicious candied almonds. Served with our famous poppyseed dressing and mini muffins. Add chicken for an additional charge.

Tropical Salad – Crisp iceberg and romaine lettuce topped with fresh sliced strawberries, Mandarin orange, pineapple tidbits, blueberries, pecans and chunks of fresh turkey breast or grilled chicken. Served with our famous poppyseed dressing and mini muffins.

Cobb Salad – Crisp iceberg and romaine lettuce topped with chunks of grilled chicken, Monterey Jack and cheddar cheese, fresh crumbled bacon, black olives, tomatoes, chopped eggs and crumbled blue cheese (optional). Served with your choice of dressing. I ask the waitperson to ask the chef to substitute extra cheddar cheese for the bacon.

Soup and Salad Combo – A bowl of our delicious homemade soup and a fresh tossed salad served with your choice of dressing.

Salad Dressing:

Our famous Sweet n' Sour Italian

Poppyseed

Honey-Dijon

Ranch

Bleu Cheese

Homemade Soups:

Our homemade soups are made fresh daily. Available by the cup or bowl.

Cream of Broccoli – Deliciously rich and creamy soup with fresh tender broccoli.

Canadian Cheese – A blend of fresh vegetables and sharp cheddar cheese combined for a real favorite!

Vegetable Beef – A rich, beefy broth filled with lots of fresh vegetables. Just like Grandma used to make!

Our Famous White Chili – A blend of white chicken meat, great white Northern beans, green chilies and Monterey Jack cheese. It's terrific!

Specialty Soup – Ask your server about our featured soup of the day.

Specialties:

Blue Owl Daily Special – A delicious home cooked meal! Ask about our daily special.

Quiche of the Day – Fresh whipped cream, eggs and cheese baked in our own tender, flaky pie crust. Served with a cup of homemade soup and a small tossed salad.

Baked Chicken Salad Pie – Tender chunks of white chicken meat, sliced water chestnuts, celery, onion, cheddar cheese and sour cream, all baked in our tender, flaky homemade crust topped with melted cheddar cheese. Served with a cup of homemade soup.

Tuesday – Meatloaf of the day.

Thursday – Chef's Special (changes weekly)

Served Every Sunday – Roast beef with Real Mashed Potatoes & other daily specials. I ask the waitperson to ask the chef to substitute a vegetable for the mashed potatoes.

Sandwiches:

All sandwiches come with your choice of small tossed salad, Hawaiian coleslaw or chips unless otherwise noted. A vegetable or a coup of soup can be added for an extra charge.

Reuben – Slices of top round corned beef grilled on marble rye with sauerkraut, Swiss cheese and Thousand Island dressing. Served with our homemade German potato salad or Fries. I ask the waitperson to ask the chef to substitute mustard for the Thousand Island dressing and to substitute a cup of soup for the potato.

Mediterranean Chicken Sandwich – Grilled chicken breast served on an asiago cheese bagel with lettuce, tomato, feta and provel cheese, pesto sauce, red onions and a creamy artichoke sauce.

Country Burger – Homemade beef patty garnished with fresh lettuce, tomato, sliced onion and pickle. Add Swiss or cheddar cheese for an additional charge.

Open Faced Roast Beef – Tender slices of top round of beef over sliced white bread and smothered with our rich brown gravy. Served with homemade mashed potatoes. I ask the waitperson to ask the chef to substitute a vegetable for the mashed potatoes.

Southern Roast Beef – Tender slices of top round of beef, hot and juicy on an onion roll smothered with grilled onions and provel cheese. Served with au jus.

BBQ Beef – Smoked beef brisket simmered in BBQ sauce and garnished with pickles and sliced onions.

Hot Roast Beef – Tender slices of top round of beef, hot and juicy, on a French roll. Served with au jus and chips. I ask the waitperson to ask the chef to substitute a vegetable for the chips.

Croissants:

Chicken Salad Croissant – Created in our own kitchen with moist, tender chicken breast, mayonnaise, crunchy celery, onions, pecans and seasoning. Served on a croissant with a cup of homemade soup.

Smoked Turkey Melt – Tender slices of smoked turkey breast and Swiss cheese melted on a croissant. Served with a cup of homemade soup.

Side orders:

Hawaiian Coleslaw

Vegetable of the Day

Fresh Fruit Cup

Dinner Salad

Homemade Pies:

Tender, flaky crusts are a must! Choose from a variety of freshly baked fruit, cream and specialty pies. Also available by the slice.

Blue Owl Creations

Chocolate Chip Pecan

Old Fashioned Pecan

Butterscotch Pecan

German Chocolate

Seasonal Pies

Fresh Strawberry

Strawberry Lovers

Apple Strudel Cheese

Bailey's Irish Cream Pie

The Blue Owl

Sweet Shoppe
Kimmswick, MO

Located next door to the Blue Owl Restaurant & Bakery, the Sweet Shop serves the same salads, sandwiches, quiches, and soups the Blue Owl Restaurant & Bakery does.

Bravo!/Brio

Chain Restaurant

Bravo!/Brio's regular menu is not listed here because it is listed in the first edition of *FROM FAT TO FABULOUS: A DIET GUIDE FOR RESTAURANT LOVERS* UNDER BRIO.

Update – Bravo!/Brio has added "The Lighter Side of Rome – Dishes Under 550 Calories" to their menu. Because I do not count calories, I eat these dishes on a day when I want a light meal.

Appetizers:

Caprese Salad – A classic with marinated tomatoes, fresh Mozzarella, basil and field greens with balsamic vinaigrette.

Italian Wedding Soup – With Chicken stock, meatballs, spinach, Parmesan, and pasta.

Salads:

Field Greens Salad – With Roma tomatoes, Feta, bacon, and Italian dressing. I ask the waitperson to ask the chef to substitute extra tomatoes for the bacon.

Chopped Salad – Chopped greens, cucumbers, red onions, tomatoes, olives, Feta cheese, and Italian dressing. I ask the waitperson to ask the chef to substitute extra chopped greens for the cucumbers.

Chopped Salad with Grilled Chicken – Chopped greens, cucumbers, red onions, tomatoes, olives, Feta cheese, and Italian dressing. I ask the waitperson to ask the chef to substitute extra red onions for the cucumbers.

Grilled Balsamic Chicken Salad – Field greens, cucumbers, red onions, Gorgonzola, strawberries, blueberries with Italian dressing. I ask the waitperson to ask the chef to substitute extra strawberries for the cucumbers.

Entrées:

Chicken Caprese – Grilled chicken layered with marinated tomatoes and Mozzarella on a bed of orzo, faro, and spinach with pesto vinaigrette.

Grilled Chicken & Vegetable Pasta – Spinach, caramelized onions, tomatoes, roasted red peppers, pesto, and fresh basil tossed with Feta and Parmesan cheeses.

Seasonal Frittata – Quiche-style frittata with fresh seasonal ingredients served warm with a side of fresh fruit.

Buffalo Wild Wings Grill & Bar

Chain Restaurant

Sharables & Sides:

Spinach Artichoke Dip – Served with warm pita chips. I do not eat the chips.

Chili Con Queso Dip – A winning blend of queso and chili served with tortilla chips. I do not eat the chips.

Side Salad

Coleslaw

Veggie Boat – Celery and carrot sticks served with a side of fat-free ranch dressing. I ask the waitperson to ask the chef for regular ranch dressing.

Savory Salads:

Honey BBQ Chicken Salad – Fresh greens, pico de gallo, a blend of cheeses, grilled chicken and BBQ ranch dressing garnished with our signature honey BBQ™ sauce.

Asian Zing® Chicken Salad – Heat meets sweet with this combination. Crisp greens, cabbage, grilled chicken and mandarin oranges garnished with our signature Asian Zing® sauce and Asian sesame dressing.

Grilled Blackened Chicken Salad – Grilled chicken with roasted garlic rub served over a fresh garden salad. Give your taste buds a thrill ride.

Grilled Chicken Salad – Seasoned, grilled chicken served over fresh greens with tomatoes, onions, a blend of cheeses and croutons. I ask the waitperson to ask the chef to substitute extra greens for the croutons.

Beefy Burgers:

Black & Bleu Burger – You should see the other burger.

Seasoned for that bayou bite, topped with bleu cheese dressing.

Cheeseburger – A true champion. Topped with admiration and your choice of American, cheddar, pepper Jack or Swiss. Add your favorite Buffalo Wild Wings sauce and create a trophy of taste. I order the burger with Swiss, cheddar or pepper Jack cheese.

Honey BBQ™ Bacon Burger – Topped with our signature Honey BBQ™ sauce, sliced cheese and bacon. Served with lettuce, tomato, and onion. I ask the waitperson to ask the chef to substitute extra tomato for the bacon.

Juicy Steak Sandwich – Between two slammer patties, a pile of juicy steak, fried onion rings, pepper Jack cheese, and your choice of Buffalo Wild Wings sauce. I ask the waitperson to ask the chef to substitute raw onion for the fried onion rings.

Satisfying Sandwiches:

Jerk Chicken Sandwich – Blackened grilled chicken breast topped with our signature Caribbean Jerk™ sauce and bleu cheese dressing.

Honey BBQ™ Bacon Chicken Sandwich – Seasoned, grilled chicken breast with crispy bacon, our signature Honey BBQ™ sauce, and sliced cheese. Go wild. I ask the waitperson to ask the chef to substitute extra cheese for the bacon.

You-Deserve-It Desserts:

Ice Cream – Ready for overtime. Dig into a scoop of frosty vanilla ice cream, showered with a drizzle of throwback of chocolate or caramel topping.

Chocolate Fudge Cake – This is a first-place finish. A big rich slice of chocolate fudge cake drizzled with chocolate sauce and served with vanilla ice cream. Yep, chocolate on top of chocolate.

Canyon Café/Sam's Café

Southwestern Grill
Chain Restaurant

Southwest Appetizers:

South Texas Tortilla Soup – Traditional southwestern soup thickened with tortillas to add a delicate corn flavor. I ask the waitperson to ask the chef to leave off the tortilla strips.

Pueblo House Salad – Fresh field greens tossed with our house made honey chipotle vinaigrette and topped with Roma tomatoes, red onions, and carrots.

Roasted Artichoke Queso Dip – A rich cheese dip flavored with pico de gallo, roasted artichokes and pepper Jack cheese. Served with flour tortillas and crisp chips. I do not eat the tortillas or the chips.

Sandwiches & Salads:

For an additional charge, add a cup of tortilla soup to any of our salads or sandwiches.

Southwest Chicken Sandwich – Adovo-grilled chicken topped with Monterey Jack and portabella mushrooms. Served on our toasted signature bun with tossed greens, chipotle mayo and crisp fries. I ask the waitperson to ask the chef to substitute grilled vegetables for the fries.

Canyon Classic Burger – Pepper Jack cheese, bacon, and our smoky BBQ sauce on a signature toasted bun with tomato and field greens. Served with crisp fries. I ask the waitperson to ask the chef to substitute grilled vegetables for the bacon and the fries.

Fajita Steak Salad – Caliente y Frio. Blackened fajita steak cooked to order and served over fresh greens tossed in red onion vinaigrette. Topped with Monterey Jack cheese and sautéed onions and peppers.

Canyon-Mex:

Chile-Rubbed Sirloin – A mild blend of herbs and spices on an 11-ounce sirloin. Fire-grilled and served with sautéed spinach and chile mashed potatoes. I ask the waitperson to ask the chef to substitute grilled vegetables for the mashed potatoes.

Carne Asada – 11-ounce fire-grilled sirloin topped with sautéed peppers, onions, mushrooms and melted Jack cheese. Served with southwest black beans, and warm flour tortillas. I ask the waitperson to ask the chef to substitute grilled vegetables for the black beans and flour tortillas.

Adovo Ribeye Steak – Fire-grilled 14-ounce Ribeye steak topped with spicy Adovo mushrooms and grated cheese. Served with chile mashed potatoes and seasonal vegetables. I ask the waitperson to ask the chef to substitute extra seasonal vegetables for the mashed potatoes.

Mex-Mex:

Fajitas – Flip & Sizzlers – Lightly marinated chicken or steak grilled to order with our unique grilled onion and pepper mix. Served with southwest rice, black beans, soft flour tortillas, and fajita toppings. I ask the waitperson to ask the chef to substitute extra grilled onions and peppers for the rice, black beans, and tortillas.

Carrabba's Italian Grill

Chain Restaurant

Cucina Casuale:

Casual Dining, Italian Style

For an extra charge you can add a soup or a side salad.

Zuppe & Insalate – Homemade Soups. Soup of the Day, Minestrone or Mama Mandola's Sicilian Chicken soup.

Side Salads – House, Italian or Caesar. For an additional charge add crumbled blue cheese. On the Caesar salad I ask the waitperson to ask the chef to substitute Italian dressing for the Caesar dressing and to leave off the croutons.

Soup & Salad – A cup of our homemade Minestrone soup served with a side Italian salad with low-fat sundried tomato vinaigrette.

Insalata Carrabba Caesar – Wood-grilled chicken in our own Caesar dressing. I ask the waitperson to ask the chef to substitute Italian dressing for the Caesar dressing and to substitute extra Romaine lettuce for the croutons.

Insalata Italian Cobb – Wood-grilled chicken, bacon, tomatoes, egg and blue cheese in vinaigrette. For an extra charge you can substitute sirloin for the chicken. I ask the waitperson to ask the chef to substitute extra tomato for the bacon.

Insalata Fiorucci – Artichoke hearts, roasted red peppers and grilled eggplant in vinaigrette, topped with hazelnut goat cheese medallion.

Signature Pasta:

All pasta dishes are served with a cup of our homemade soup or a side salad. Any signature pasta may be made with whole grain spaghetti.

Spaghetti – Topped with pomodoro sauce. Meatballs or meat

sauce is an extra charge. I eat spaghetti on a reward night.

Penne Franco – Mushrooms, sundried tomatoes, artichoke hearts and black olives, in garlic and oil with ricotta salata cheese. You can add chicken for an additional charge. I eat Penne Franco on a reward night.

Pasta Carrabba – Fettuccine Alf redo with grilled chicken, sautéed mushrooms and peas. I eat this pasta on a reward night.

Stuffed Pasta:

Chicken & Spinach Cannelloni – Chicken, spinach, garlic, fresh herbs, fontina and Romano cheese, topped with pomodoro and cream sauce. I eat this cannelloni on a reward night.

Marsala:

Topped with mushrooms, prosciutto and our Lombardo Marsala. I ask the waitperson to ask the chef to substitute extra mushrooms for the prosciutto.

Chicken

Sirloin

Veal

Classics & Combinations:

The Johnny" – Sirloin Marsala and Chicken Bryan

Veal Piccata – Sautéed, topped with lemon butter sauce.

Wood-Burning Grill:

Chicken Bryan – Topped with goat cheese, sundried tomatoes and basil lemon butter sauce.

Grilled Chicken – Basted with olive oil and herbs.

Filet Marsala

Dolci:

Ask your server about our seasonal dessert selection.

<u>Sogno Di Cioccolata "Chocolate Dream</u> – A rich fudge brownie brushed with Kahlua, with chocolate mousse, whipped cream and homemade chocolate sauce.

<u>Tiramisu</u> – Lady Fingers dipped in liqueur laced espresso, layered with sweetened mascarpone. Myer's Rum and chocolate shavings.

<u>John Cole</u> – Vanilla ice cream with caramel sauce and roasted cinnamon rum pecans.

Charleston's

Oklahoma City, Norman, & Edmond, OK

Starters:

Creamed Spinach Artichoke Dip – In a parmesan cream sauce with fresh tortilla chips.

Soup Calendar:

Monday – Roasted Tomato and Vegetable.

Thursday – Tortilla. I ask the waitperson to ask the chef to leave off the chips.

Saturday – Chef's Choice

Sunday – Beef & Vegetable.

Sides:

Seasonal Vegetable

Coleslaw

Burgundy Mushrooms

Burgers & Sandwiches:

Choose coleslaw or a cup of soup.

Cheeseburger – Cheddar, lettuce, tomato, onion, pickles and mayonnaise.

Reuben – Sliced corned beef, sauerkraut, Swiss cheese, and Thousand Island dressing. I ask the waitperson to ask the chef to substitute mustard for the Thousand Island dressing.

Famous French Dip – Thinly sliced prime rib. Served on a toasted French roll.

Salads:

Dressings: Bleu Cheese, Creamy Garlic, Herbal Vinaigrette, Honey-Mustard.

Spinach & Chicken Waldorf Salad – Spinach and field greens, grilled chicken, raisins, apples, strawberries, egg, spiced pecans, sharp cheddar, sweet bacon vinaigrette. I ask the waitperson to substitute bleu cheese or honey-mustard for the sweet bacon vinaigrette.

Walt's Champagne Chicken Salad – Mixed greens, pineapple, dates, feta, strawberries, spiced pecans, sunflower seeds, croutons, and champagne vinaigrette. I ask the waitperson to ask the chef to substitute extra sunflower seeds for the croutons.

Soup and Salad – House-made soup of the day served with a house salad.

Chicken:

Enchilada Plate – Corn tortilla filled with grilled chicken, Monterey Jack, enchilada red sauce and served with sour cream, guacamole and vine-ripe tomatoes. I ask the waitperson to ask the chef to serve the enchilada open faced and to substitute extra tomatoes for the guacamole.

Oven Roasted Chicken – (limited availability) One-half herb-roasted chicken served with garlic mashed potatoes and smokehouse baked beans. I ask the waitperson to ask the chef to substitute the seasonal vegetable and burgundy mushrooms for the mashed potatoes and smokehouse baked beans.

Parmesan Crusted Chicken – Seasoned in a parmesan, walnut and pecan crust. Topped with marinara on a bed of angel hair pasta. Served with a pear tomato, mozzarella and red onion herbal salad. I ask the waitperson to ask the chef to substitute the seasonal vegetable for the angel hair pasta.

Chicken Piccata – Pan seared, tossed with artichokes, asparagus and tomatoes in a lemon caper butter sauce on angel hair pasta with seasonal vegetables. I ask the waitperson to ask the chef to substitute extra asparagus for the angel hair pasta.

Steaks & Prime Rib:

Top Sirloin – 10 oz. Hardwood grilled with baked potato and a house salad. I ask the waitperson to ask the chef to substitute the burgundy mushrooms for the baked potato.

Center Cut Filet – 7 oz. Hardwood grilled, with baked potato and a house salad. I ask the waitperson to ask the chef to substitute the seasonal vegetables for the baked potato.

Prime Rib – (available after 4:00pm) Seasoned and slow roasted with garlic mashed potatoes and a house salad. Available in 10 oz. or 14 oz. I ask the waitperson to ask the chef to substitute asparagus or broccoli for the garlic mashed potatoes.

Cheeseburger Cheeseburger

Chain Restaurant

Invent your own cheeseburgers, shakes, wraps, sandwiches, salads, desserts, and more!

Sauces:

Creamy Cheese – Cheese lover's delight.

Zesty Horseradish – Not too hot.

reamy Jalapeno – Has a little kick.

Garden Vegetable – Refreshing.

Invent Your Salad!

Each salad includes a generous spring mix of chopped Romaine and a collection of fresh baby greens with your choice of dressings. Combine any of the FREE TOPPINGS and create your own favorite.

Combination Grilled Portobello and Grilled Chicken Salad

Grilled Chicken Breast Salad

Grilled Portobello Mushroom Salad

Turkey Burger Salad

Cheeseburger Salad

Salad Lover's Salad – A generous salad made of mixed greens.

Side Salad – Mixed greens with black olives, shredded Jack and cheddar, grape tomatoes and garlic croutons. I ask the waitperson to ask the chef to leave off the croutons.

Salad Dressings:

Bleu cheese, ranch, Greek, honey mustard, oil & vinegar, balsamic vinaigrette, fat free raspberry vinaigrette, low cal Italian.

Invent Your Cheeseburger!

Free cheese & toppings for Burgers, Wraps, Sandwiches, Platters, and Salads. Over 8,721,000 Burger Combinations.

Our Famous Pounder Burger – Actually a huge 20 ounces!

The Delirious Burger – 3/4 lb. (14 ounces)

The Serious Burger – 1/2 lb. (10 ounces)

The Semi-Serious Burger Everybody's favorite! 1/3 lb. (7 ounces)

The Classic Burger 1/4 lb. (5.5 ounces)

The Turkey Burger

In a hurry? Please remember, we are not fast food. We cook everything to order.

Pick one cheese. Any cheese:

Swiss cheese, Cheddar cheese, Provolone cheese, Bleu cheese, Provel cheese, Pepper Jack cheese, Feta cheese, Smoked Gouda cheese, or Havarti Cheese.

Add specialty toppings for just a little more:

Sautéed mushrooms, Sautéed onions, chili grilled or Portobello mushroom.

Free Toppings!

Lettuce, Tomato, Onion, Pickle, Mayonnaise, 1000 island dressing, 2 onion rings, Bar-B-Que sauce, Cavenders Greek seasoning, Chipotle mayo, Chopped garlic, Coleslaw, Grey poupon, Honey mustard, Horseradish, Horseradish sauce, Relish, Salsa, Pineapple, Ranch dressing Roasted Red peppers, Sun dried tomatoes Teriyaki Sauce. FOR SALADS ONLY Baby carrots, Bleu Crumbles, Dried cranberries, Feta Cheese, Grape tomatoes, Green peppers, Jack/cheddar mix, Mushrooms, Parmesan cheese, Sunflower seeds.

Invent Your Platter . . .

Your choice of cheese & toppings, sautéed onions, and choice of side salad or coleslaw.

Angus Burger Platter - Fresh, never frozen 10 oz. patty.

Chicken Breast Platter - Succulent grilled chicken breast.

Portobello Platter – A hearty portion of Portobello mushroom.

Turkey Burger Platter – We give you all the choices.

Invent Your Shake!

Over 1,285,000 Flavor combinations!

Almond, Amaretto, Cherry, Chocolate, Chocolate Cherry, Chocolate Chip, Hazelnut, Peach, Peach Mango, Pina Colada, Root Beer, Strawberry, and Vanilla.

City Coffee House & Creperie

Clayton, MO

Crepes:

Made with white flour or 100% organic & gluten-free. Buckwheat flour is available for an additional charge.

Cheese – Cheddar, Swiss, Havarti, Mozzarella or Pepper Jack. Brie is available for an additional charge.

Egg & Cheese – Egg and cheese and your choice of chicken or turkey.

BLT – Bacon, fresh spinach, mozzarella cheese, marinated tomatoes, green onions with our house dressing. I ask the waitperson to ask the chef to substitute turkey for the bacon.

Brittany – Honey ham, fresh asparagus, Havarti cheese and fresh spinach with Hollandaise sauce. I ask the waitperson to ask the chef to substitute turkey for the ham.

Fiesta – Grilled chicken, green chilies, red onion, fresh spinach, with mozzarella and cheddar cheese and your choice of sauce. Southwest Ranch or chili verde.

Florentine – Creamed spinach, fresh tomatoes, cheddar cheese with Hollandaise sauce.

Mediterranean Vegetable – Zucchini, fresh mushrooms, roasted red peppers, artichoke hearts, tomatoes, red onion, fresh spinach, mozzarella cheese and olive oil.

Mont Blanc – Grilled chicken, fresh mushrooms mozzarella cheese, red onion with mushroom cream sauce.

Provence – French brie and walnuts, garnished with red grapes and strawberries. I ask the waitperson to ask the chef to substitute extra strawberries for the grapes.

Santa Fe – Chorizo Pepper Jack, avocado, tomato, cilantro, red onion, fresh spinach with Juan's house-made rojo sauce topped with avocado-sour cream sauce. I ask the waitperson to ask the chef to substitute extra tomato for the avocado.

Shady Oak – Grilled chicken, fresh spinach, Havarti cheese, marinated tomatoes and green onions with our house-made honey Dijon dressing.

Shaw Park – Turkey, fresh spinach, Havarti cheese, roasted red peppers with house dressing.

St. Louis – Grilled chicken, artichoke and parmesan cheese filling and fresh spinach.

Tropicana – Grilled chicken, honey ham, pineapple, mozzarella cheese, fresh spinach with home-made honey-Dijon dressing. I ask the waitperson to ask the chef to substitute extra spinach for the ham.

Tuscany – Classic Italian pesto, mozzarella cheese, fresh basil, fresh tomatoes, roasted red peppers and spinach.

Veggie – Broccoli, carrots, fresh mushrooms, fresh spinach, mozzarella cheese, roasted red peppers, marinated tomatoes and green onions with house dressing.

Dessert Crepes:

Apple-Cinnamon & Brown Sugar

Banana-Sour Cream & Brown Sugar

Plain topped with Brown Sugar

Strawberry Jam topped with Powdered Sugar

Fresh Seasonal Fruit topped with Whipped Cream & Powdered Sugar

Chocolate (Nutella) Crepes

Freedom – Strawberries, Blueberries and Crème Fraiche

Mon Cheri Amor – Sweet cream cheese and cherry filling

Monte Carlo – Strawberries, coconut & pecans with Manjar Blanco Sauce

Raspberry Beret – Fresh raspberries & white chocolate

Quiche:

Served with freshly baked baguette.

Quiche du Jour

Quiche with a cup of soup.

Quiche with Market Salad or a side salad.

Quiche with half a sandwich.

Soups & Salads:

All soups & salads are served with a freshly baked baguette.

Side Salad (Garden)

Soup du Jour

Salad Combo – Chicken salad with Market Salad or Side Salad.

Pick 2 Combo – Cup of soup, half sandwich or small salad.

On Combo or Pick 2, Chef Salad, Chicken Caesar, Ann's Green Gable or Vineyard Chopped Salads have an additional charge.

Ann's Green Gable – Romaine lettuce, fresh spinach, mandarin oranges strawberries, red onions, and walnuts crumbled bacon & grilled chicken with poppyseed dressing. I ask the waitperson to ask the chef to substitute extra strawberries for the bacon.

Chef Salad – Romaine lettuce, tomatoes, cucumbers, shredded carrots, red onions, turkey, ham, mozzarella cheese, hard-boiled egg & house-made croutons. Dressings: Bleu cheese, Balsamic Vinaigrette, House, Italian, Honey Dijon, Poppyseed, Raspberry vinaigrette, and Red Wine Vinaigrette.

Caesar Salad – Romaine lettuce tossed with grilled chicken, roasted red peppers, artichoke hearts, red onions, parmesan, house-made croutons & Caesar dressing. I ask the waitperson to ask the chef to leave off the croutons and to substitute bleu cheese dressing for the Caesar dressing.

Vineyard Chopped Salad – Romaine lettuce, grilled chicken, bacon, avocado, eggs, tomatoes, red onions & bleu cheese tossed with Red Wine Vinaigrette. I ask the waitperson to ask the chef to substitute extra tomatoes and red onions for the bacon and avocado.

Market Salad – Fresh spinach, pineapple, grapes, mandarin oranges, strawberries, apples, bleu cheese with poppyseed dressing and garnished with seasonal fruits. I ask the waitperson to ask the chef to substitute extra strawberries for the grapes.

Stuffed Tomato – with chicken salad.

Sandwiches:

Freshly Baked Turkey – Turkey breast, fresh spinach, red onion, Havarti cheese & our house-made apple salsa.

Mike's Chicken Salad – All white meat chicken, celery, grapes & green onion mixed with Mike's famous house-made dressing.

Veggie – Fresh spinach, tomatoes, cucumbers, red peppers, mushrooms, red onion, Havarti cheese & our house-made dressing. I ask the waitperson to ask the chef to substitute extra tomatoes for the cucumbers.

Colton's Steak House & Grill

Chain Restaurant

Appetizers:

Spinach Artichoke Dip – Creamy mozzarella and parmesan cheese blended with spinach, artichokes, and minced garlic. Served with tortilla chips. I do not eat the tortilla chips.

Soup of the Day

Favorites:

All items below include homemade yeast rolls and a side of your choice. Add a house or Caesar salad for an additional charge. I do not eat the yeast rolls.

Colton's "Loaded" Chicken – A juicy grilled chicken breast covered in sautéed mushrooms, bacon, green onions, and a blend of cheeses. Served with honey mustard sauce. I ask the waitperson to ask the chef to leave off the bacon.

Mesquite Grilled Chicken – A boneless chicken breast, mesquite grilled and served on a bed of rice pilaf. I ask the waitperson to substitute steamed vegetables for the rice.

Hawaiian Chicken – A boneless chicken breast, marinated in a blend of teriyaki sauce, pineapple juice, and special seasonings. Served on a bed of rice. I ask the waitperson to substitute steamed vegetables for the rice.

Steak & Rib Dinners:

Our aged Mesquite grilled steak & rib dinners include a house or Caesar salad, homemade yeast rolls, and or side of your choice. On Caesar salads I ask the waitperson to ask the chef to leave off the croutons and to substitute bleu cheese dressing for the Caesar dressing.

Sirloin – 6 oz., 9 oz. or 12 oz.

Filet Mignon – 8 oz. wrapped in bacon. I ask the waitperson to ask the chef to prepare my filet without the bacon.

Hawaiian Ribeye – Marinated in our special Hawaiian seasonings and garnished with grilled pineapple.

Del Rio Ribeye – Rubbed with bold Southwest spices, topped with ancho chipotle butter, and Onion Tanglers. I ask the waitperson to ask the chef to substitute grilled or sautéed onions for the Onion Tanglers.

T-Bone 18 oz. – J.T.'s largest steak!

New York Strip 12 oz.

Sirloin Tips – With sautéed peppers and onions.

Chopped Sirloin 12 oz. – With peppers and onions. Topped with Onion Tanglers. . I ask the waitperson to ask the chef to substitute grilled or sautéed onions for the Onion Tanglers

Salads & Pasta:

Served with a basket of homemade yeast rolls. I do not eat the yeast rolls.

Salad Dressings – Your choice of dressings includes Colton's Homemade House dressing, Italian, Hidden Valley Ranch, Spicy Ranch, Bleu Cheese, Honey Mustard, and Balsamic Vinaigrette. I do not use the fat-free salad dressings.

Mesquite Grilled Chicken Salad – Grilled chicken strips served on a bed of fresh mixed greens, shredded cheese, diced tomatoes, sliced egg, shredded carrots, croutons, and purple onion. I ask the waitperson to ask the chef to leave off the croutons.

Southwest Chicken Salad – Grilled chicken strips blackened and served on a bed of fresh mixed greens, diced tomatoes, and black bean corn salsa, topped with thinly sliced tortilla chips. Served with ranch dressing. I ask the waitperson to ask the chef to substitute extra tomatoes for the black bean corn salsa and the tortilla chips.

Grilled Sirloin Salad – Strips of mesquite grilled sirloin steak served over fresh mixed greens, shredded cheese, diced tomatoes, sliced egg, shredded carrots, croutons, and purple onion. I ask the waitperson to ask the chef to leave off the croutons.

Caesar Salad – A Texas-sized portion of romaine lettuce and croutons tossed in our special Caesar dressing. Topped with purple onion, sliced egg, and parmesan cheese. Grilled chicken can be added for an additional charge. I ask the waitperson to ask the chef to leave off the croutons and to substitute bleu cheese dressing for the Caesar dressing.

Texas House Salad – House salad with fresh mixed greens, shredded cheese, diced tomatoes, sliced egg, shredded carrots, purple onion, croutons, and diced smoked bacon. I ask the waitperson to ask the chef to substitute extra diced tomatoes for the bacon and croutons.

Soup & Salad – A steaming bowl of either of our great soups and a dinner salad or a Caesar salad.

Burgers & Sandwiches:

Colton's burgers are made fresh with a half- pound of fresh ground beef and seasoned with our special spices. All sandwiches and burgers are served with your choice of side.

J.T.'s Charbroiled Lonesome Burger – A juicy charbroiled burger served with lettuce, tomato, pickles and onion.

Mesquite Grilled Chicken Sandwich – A grilled chicken breast served with lettuce and tomato.

Deluxe Grilled Chicken Sandwich – A tender grilled chicken breast topped with Swiss cheese and strips of bacon. I ask the waitperson to substitute tomato for the bacon strips.

Sides:

Steamed Veggies

Sautéed Mushrooms

Green Beans

Desserts:

Chocolate Sin-Station – Our scrumptious, chewy brownie with brownie with walnuts crowned with ice cream, hot fudge, whipped cream, and a cherry.

Bread Pudding – Homemade bread pudding baked to perfection served warm with pecan praline sauce and topped with vanilla ice cream.

Cooperage

Albuquerque, NM

Lunch:
Soup & Salad Bar:

Our reputation and success over the years can be partly attributed to our famous Soup & Salad Bar. All our delicious soups and salads are prepared fresh daily here at the Cooperage. Make a meal from the Soup & Salad Bar. Or have it with your lunch entrée.

Sandwiches:

Prime Rib Sandwich – A generous portion of prime rib cut to order and served on an open faced croissant with steak fries. I ask the waitperson to ask the chef to substitute the steamed vegetables for the steak fries.

Green Chile Ginza Sandwich – A grilled Hawaiian chicken breast topped with green chili, Swiss cheese and a pineapple ring on a hoagie roll. Served with potato chips. I do not eat the potato chips.

The Lobo – Grilled turkey with Swiss cheese and green chili on a hoagie roll or pita bread. Served with potato chips. I do not eat the potato chips.

Philadelphia Steak Sandwich – Shaved choice beef grilled with sautéed bell peppers, onions and mushrooms on a hoagie roll topped with melted Swiss cheese. Served with potato chips. I do not eat the potato chips.

Steaks:

Steak Ranchero – U.S.D.A. Choice top sirloin broiled to order and covered with green chili and cheddar cheese. Served with steak fries. I ask the waitperson to ask the chef to substitute steamed vegetables for the steak fries.

Top Sirloin Steak – U.S.D.A. Choice top sirloin served with

garlic toast and steak fries. I ask the waitperson to ask the chef to substitute steamed vegetables for the steak fries.

Prime Rib:

It's our specialty. Enjoy grain fed, Nebraska prime beef, roasted to perfection. Served with au jus and creamed horseradish, steak fries and oven fresh bread. I ask the waitperson to ask the chef to substitute steamed vegetables for the steak fries.

Seafood & Chicken:

Grilled Hawaiian Chicken – A tender marinated boneless breast of chicken topped with a pineapple ring and served on a bed of seasoned rice with a side of teriyaki sauce. I ask the waitperson to ask the chef to substitute steamed vegetables for the rice.

Chicken con Queso – A boneless breast of chicken wrapped around Monterey Jack cheese and green chili; lightly breaded and deep fried to a golden brown. Covered with chili con queso and served with seasoned rice. I ask the waitperson to ask the chef to substitute grilled chicken for the breaded and deep fried chicken and to substitute steamed vegetables for the rice.

Burgers:

Our made fresh daily 1/2 pound burgers are broiled to perfection and served on a fresh bun with lettuce, tomatoes, onions and pickles. Includes steak fries. On all burgers I ask the waitperson to ask the chef to substitute steamed vegetables for the steak fries.

Copper Burger with Cheese

Mushroom Swiss Burger

South of the Border Burger – Covered with melted cheddar cheese and topped with green chili and guacamole. I ask the waitperson to ask the chef to substitute extra tomato slices for the guacamole.

Buffalo Burger – Extra lean (6 oz.) heart healthy burger with a unique flavor from the great outdoors.

More Favorites:

BBQ Bits of Beef – A casserole dish of tender bits of beef in a tangy BBQ sauce. This has been a Cooperage favorite for over 30 years! Served with steak fries or rice. I ask the waitperson to ask the chef to substitute steamed vegetables for the steak fries or rice.

Chopped Sirloin Supreme – A generous 10 oz. portion of fresh ground chuck broiled to perfection and smothered with a mushroom-onion wine sauce. Served with steak fries or seasoned rice. I ask the waitperson to ask the chef to substitute steamed vegetables for the steak fries or rice.

Dinner:

Our reputation and success over the years can be partly attributed to our famous Soup & Salad Bar. All our delicious soups and salads are prepared fresh daily here at the Cooperage. Make a meal from the Soup & Salad Bar. Or have it with your dinner entrée.

Prime Rib:

It's our specialty. Enjoy grain fed, Nebraska prime beef, roasted to perfection. Served with au jus and creamed horseradish, choice of potato, seasoned rice or steak fries. Includes oven fresh bread and unlimited trips to our bountiful soup and salad bar. I ask the waitperson to ask the chef to substitute steamed vegetables for the steak fries, potato, or rice.

Standard Cut

Managers Cut

Cooper Cut

Steaks & Chops:

From the grill . . . we proudly serve only U.S.D.A. choice & prime beef specifically aged and cut on the premises daily.

Dinner entrées include unlimited trips to the bountiful soup & salad bar, oven fresh bread & your choice of rice, baked potato or steak fries. On all steaks and chops I ask the waitperson to ask the chef to substitute steamed vegetables for the rice, baked potato, or steak fries.

Cooper Cut Top Sirloin – Feast on the best 10 oz. top sirloin in Albuquerque. It's tender, it's tasty and it's grilled to perfection.

Lamb Chops Rosemary – Marinated in a wonderful mustard-herb blend and grilled to your liking.

Steak Ranchero – Top sirloin smothered with green chili and cheese.

Teriyaki Top Sirloin – Marinated in the perfect teriyaki sauce and grilled to your order.

New York Strip – A 13-oz. cut, grilled to order.

Steak & Bake – Famous 1/2 pound top sirloin served with baked potato.

Buffalo Steak – An extra lean, 1/2 pound New York cut of Wyoming-raised buffalo. It's lean and heart smart.

Chopped Sirloin Supreme – 10 oz. of fresh ground beef smothered with burgundy-mushroom-onion sauce.

Filet Mignon – (bacon wrapped) Cut from the tenderloin. It's lean and tender! I ask the waitperson to ask the chef to prepare my filet mignon without the bacon.

Petite Filet Mignon – (bacon wrapped) Perfect for the smaller appetite. I ask the waitperson to ask the chef to prepare my filet mignon without the bacon.

Dress up your steak with mushrooms sautéed in butter, garlic and wine or fresh grilled onions or steamed vegetables for an additional charge.

First Watch

Chain Restaurant

Omelets:

Served with either dressed greens or fresh, seasoned potatoes and an English muffin. Cholesterol/fat-free eggs or egg whites may be substituted at no additional charge. I order the fresh greens.

Killer Cajun® - Spicy Cajun all natural white-meat chicken breast with house roasted Crimini mushrooms, onions and Monterey Jack. Served with a side of Santa Fe sauce.

Greek Fetish® - Roasted red peppers, spinach, onions with feta and black olives.

C'est La Vie – House-roasted zucchini, onions and tomatoes with herbed goat cheese.

Veg'd Out™ - House-roasted Crimini mushrooms, zucchini, onions, tomatoes and broccoli with cheddar and Monterey Jack.

The Forager – House-roasted Crimini mushrooms and tomatoes with fresh herbs, mozzarella and Swiss.

Swiss Room - Ham, house-roasted Crimini mushrooms and onions with fresh herbs and Swiss. I ask the waitperson to ask the chef to substitute extra mushrooms for the ham.

First Watch® Eggs-clusives:

Caps, Etc® - House-roasted Crimini mushrooms topped with melted cheddar and Monterey Jack. Served with two fresh eggs any style and an English muffin. I ask the waitperson to substitute extra cheddar for the English muffin.

Turkey Chive Crepegg® - A thin crepe layered with eggs, turkey, spinach, house-roasted onions and Monterey Jack. Topped with diced tomatoes, chives and hollandaise. Served with an English muffin. I ask the waitperson to ask the chef to substitute extra tomatoes for the English muffin.

Fresh Spring Mix Salads:

Pecan Dijon® - All-natural white-meat chicken breast, bacon, avocado, pecans, tomato and carrots with cheddar and Monterey Jack. Drizzled with warm honey Dijon dressing. Available as a 2 for You. I ask the waitperson to ask the chef to substitute extra tomatoes and greens for the bacon and avocado.

No. 5 Asian – All-natural white-meat chicken breast, crispy wontons, sliced almonds, fresh cilantro and carrots with sesame Asian dressing. I ask the waitperson to ask the chef to substitute extra greens for the crispy wontons. Also available as a 2 for You.

Fruity Chicken – Our all-natural white-meat chicken salad served with baby spinach, tomato, seasonal fruit and poppyseed dressing.

Santa Fe – Cajun all-natural white-meat chicken breast, house-roasted Crimini mushrooms, tomato, avocado, house-made ciabatta croutons. Cheddar and Monterey Jack with Santa Fe dressing. Also available as a 2 for You. I ask the waitperson to ask the chef to substitute extra tomatoes and mushrooms for the avocado and ciabatta croutons.

2 for You®:

1/2 sandwich + 1/4 salad. * 1/2 sandwich + cup of soup * 1/ 4 salad + cup of soup

Choose two half portions of some of our lunch favorites. Look for the 2 for You®.

Sandwiches:

Served with dressed greens or a bowl of hot soup.

Chicken Salad Melt – All-natural white-meat chicken salad made with apples, raisins and celery served open-faced on grilled multigrain. Topped with tomato and melted Monterey Jack.

Grilled Turkey – Turkey, bacon, tomato and Monterey Jack with ranch dressing on grilled sourdough. Also available on the 2 for You. I ask the waitperson to ask the chef to substitute extra Monterey Jack for the bacon.

Baja Turkey Burger – A lean white-meat Turkey patty with avocado, lettuce, house-made salsa, mayo and pepper Jack on a grilled wheat bun. I ask the waitperson to ask the chef to substitute extra pepper Jack for the avocado.

Reuben Corned beef or turkey on rye with Thousand Island, sauerkraut and Swiss. Also available on the 2 for You. I ask the waitperson to ask the chef to substitute mustard for the Thousand Island dressing.

Beefeater Roast beef, tomato, cheddar and Monterey Jack on grilled Parmesan-crusted sourdough. Horseradish sauce on the side. Also available on the 2 for You.

Pesto Roast Beef – Roast beef, roasted tomatoes, spinach and Swiss with pickled red onion and a basil pesto spread on grilled sourdough.

Chicken Palermo – Grilled all-natural white-meat chicken, sliced tomato, onion, pepperoncini and mozzarella with basil pesto mayo on artisan ciabatta.

2 for You®

Lunch that's twice as nice. Chose two from the following: 1/2 sandwich * 1/4 salad * cup of soup.

Sandwiches

Reuben

Grilled Turkey

Beefeater

Salads

House

No. 5 Asian

Pecan Dijon

Santa Fe

Soups

Soup of the Day

Tomato Basil

Sides and Small Plates:

Bowl of Soup – Tomato Basil or Soup of the Day

Fruit Bowl – Filled with fresh seasonal fruit

Turkey Sausage

Five Star Burgers

Chain Restaurant

Burgers:

Our 100% Angus beef is fresh, all natural, and antibiotic free from Harris Ranch. We grind and form our burgers daily, grill to your taste, and serve on a toasted brioche bun.

5 Star Burger – Gorgonzola cheese and Applewood smoked bacon. I ask the waitperson to ask the chef to substitute extra cheese for the bacon.

Old Timer – Tomato, lettuce, onion, pickle, and condiments.

Taos Burger – Crispy green chile, BBQ sauce, and cheddar cheese.

Green Chile Cheeseburger – Green chile, pepper Jack cheese, and green chile mayo.

Bison Burger – Colorado bison and grilled onions. Grilled medium.

Additional Toppings:

For an additional charge –

Aged Cheddar

Pepper Jack

Gorgonzola

Crispy Green Chili

Wild Mushrooms

Swiss Cheese

Smoked Provolone

Grilled Onions

Specialty Burgers & Sandwiches:

5 Star Turkey Burger – Sage, peach or cranberry chutney, red onion, and mayo. I order the cranberry chutney.

Green Chile Chicken – All natural chicken breast, green chile, pepper Jack cheese, and green chile mayo.

Lamb Burger – Greek Tzatzki sauce, lettuce and tomato.

Entrées:

Harris Ranch Hamburger Steak – 12 oz. of our Angus beef, charbroiled, Gorgonzola cream, caramelized onions, French fries, and grilled vegetables. I ask the waitperson to ask the chef to substitute extra grilled vegetables for the French fries.

Salads:

Shanghai Chicken – Asian and field greens, almonds, green onions, water chestnuts, crispy wonton noodles, sprouts, sesame seeds, and Thai peanut dressing. I ask the waitperson to ask the chef to substitute extra field greens for the crispy wonton noodles.

Spinach – Organic baby spinach, Gorgonzola, strawberry slices, shaved sweet onion, glazed walnuts, dried cranberries, and creamy lemon dressing.

Chop Chop Chicken – Diced all natural chicken, mixed lettuces, sweet corn, black beans, cheddar cheese, slivered almonds, cilantro, red pepper, celery, green onion, cucumber, tortilla chips, ranch dressing, and BBQ drizzle. I ask the waitperson to ask the chef to substitute extra lettuce, red pepper, and almonds for the corn, beans, cucumber, and tortilla chips.

Vegetable Chop - Field greens, red pepper, green onions, sweet corn, celery, golden raisins, sunflower seeds, cucumber, balsamic vinaigrette dressing. For an additional charge you can add Gorgonzola crumbles. I ask the waitperson to ask the chef to substitute extra field greens, red pepper, and green onions for the corn and cucumbers.

<u>Side Green Salad</u> – Side salad with any burger, sandwich or entrée.

For an additional charge you can add all natural chicken breast or Harris Ranch beef burger to any salad.

Hayashi

Albuquerque, NM and Lubbock, TX

Teriyaki:

Broiled with onions, broccoli, carrots, and teriyaki sauce, served with soup, salad and white rice.

Chicken – White meat chicken

Beef

Beef Negimaki – Broiled scallion wrapped in thinly sliced beef

Hibachi Combination Dinners:

All entrées are served with clear soup, a house salad, grilled noodles and two piece shrimp appetizer. My husband eats my shrimp appetizer and noodles.

New York Strip and Chicken

Hibachi Filet Mignon and Chicken

Hibachi Dinners:

All entrées are served with clear soup, a house salad, grilled noodles and two piece shrimp appetizer. My husband eats my shrimp appetizer and noodles.

Hibachi Vegetables – Sautéed fresh garden vegetables served with hibachi fried rice.

Hibachi Beef Teriyaki – Teriyaki style hibachi Angus steak mixed with sautéed onions, served with sautéed fresh garden vegetables and hibachi fried rice.

Hibachi Chicken – Hibachi grilled chicken breast served with our hibachi vegetables and fried rice.

Hibachi Steak – Hand cut Angus New York strip lightly seasoned and grilled to perfection, served with sautéed fresh garden vegetables and hibachi fried rice.

<u>Hibachi Filet Mignon</u> – Hand cut filet mignon grilled to your specification and served with fresh hibachi vegetables and fried rice.

Helen Fitzgerald's

St. Louis, MO

Appetizers:

Spinach Artichoke Dip – Our award-winning blend of fresh spinach, artichoke, mayonnaise, parmesan and cream cheeses baked to perfection. Served with our homemade potato chips or pita chips. I do not eat the chips.

Vegie Spring Rolls – Served with pineapple salsa.

Fresh Salads and Soups:

Soup of the Day – Made fresh daily, asks your server for today's choice.

Chili – Paul's famous award-winning recipe.

Fitzgerald's House Salad – A mixture of iceberg and romaine lettuce with sliced red onions, diced red peppers, homemade croutons, shredded provel cheese and your choice of dressing. I ask the waitperson to ask the chef to substitute extra romaine lettuce for the croutons.

Real Estate Salad – Same as our house salad plus ham, salami, turkey, and your choice of dressing. I ask the waitperson to ask the chef to substitute extra turkey for the ham.

Shamrock Chicken Walnut Salad – Large dinner salad plus strips of charbroiled chicken breast, toasted walnuts and your choice of dressing.

Cobb Salad – House salad stacked with chicken, tomato, egg, mandarin orange, bleu cheese crumbles and your choice of dressing.

Taco Salad – Taco shell filled with lettuce, seasoned beef, cheddar cheese, onion, tomato, black olive and served with salsa ranch dressing. I do not eat the taco shell.

Shamrock Dinner Salad – Iceberg lettuce, homemade croutons,

shredded provel cheese and your choice of dressing. I ask the waitperson to ask the chef to substitute extra lettuce for the croutons.

Dinner Only:

4:00pm to closing.

Helen Fitzgerald's Pasta and Irish Entrées:

Served with choice of soup or salad.

Corned Beef and Cabbage – An Irish tradition that speaks for itself.

Irish Beef Stew – Helen Fitzgerald's famous homemade recipe of tender beef and fresh veggies.

Burgers:

All burgers come with fries or coleslaw. All Helen Fitzgerald's burgers are handmade from USDA sirloin that is fresh ground daily. Each burger is ¾ lb. and carefully charbroiled according to your liking and served on a large bun with lettuce, tomato, onion and pickle slices. I always order the coleslaw.

Old Fashion Hamburger – This burger speaks for itself.

Gourmet Burger – Bleu cheese and sautéed mushrooms.

Rich's Special – Sautéed onions, mushrooms and cheddar cheese.

Fitzgerald Frisco Melt – Swiss and provel cheese on grilled sourdough with 1000 Thousand Island dressing. I ask the waitperson to ask the chef to substitute mustard for the Thousand Island dressing.

Cajun Burger – Spiced with Cajun seasonings and topped with sautéed onions, green peppers and pepper Jack cheese.

Sandwiches:

All sandwiches served with choice of fries, chips or

homemade coleslaw and a big kosher pickle. Cheese is available for an additional charge. I always order the coleslaw.

 Lean Corned Beef Piled on Marble Rye – Served with horseradish on the side.

Reuben – You haven't tasted a Reuben until you've tasted one from an Irish kitchen.

Roast Beef on French Bread – Our top round beef sliced fresh and served on French bread.

Grilled Chicken Breast – On a whole wheat bun with bacon, lettuce and tomato. Served with mayo on the side. I ask the waitperson to ask the chef to substitute extra tomato for the bacon.

Cajun Chicken Breast – Mildly seasoned and topped with sautéed onions and green peppers on a large fresh Kaiser bun.

Steak & Chicken Entrées:

All dinner entrées are served with Helen's salad or soup, and choice of potato or vegetable. I always order the vegetable.

8 oz. Filet Mignon – (choice of traditional or peppered) A thick cut of absolutely the most tender corn fed Midwest beef you have ever enjoyed. Charbroiled and seasoned to your satisfaction. It will melt in your mouth.

8 oz. Steak Provel – Charbroiled center cut strip steak smothered with provel cheese and mushrooms.

Glazed 12 oz. New York Strip – Center Cut strip steak seasoned to perfection and charbroiled to your liking.

Chicken Provel – Pan fried chicken breast smothered with melted provel cheese and mushrooms. Outstanding!

Low Cal Chicken Breast – Seasoned with lemon pepper, charbroiled and served with vegetable and salad.

Jack Daniels Glazed Chicken Breast – Grilled chicken breast, glazed wih homemade Jack Daniels sauce.

Desserts:

Grandma's Favorite – A delicious melt in your mouth brownie topped with vanilla ice cream, hot fudge, and hot caramel, crushed walnuts and shipped cream.

Lunch Specialties:

Served from 11:00am to 4:00pm.

Same as dinner specials but in smaller portions.

Blue Plate – The Chef's special made daily just like mom used to make. Ask your server.

Lunch Special – Something new and special every day.

Hoffbrau Steaks

Texas Chain Restaurant

Hoffbrau Signature Steaks:

Our steaks are USDA Certified corn fed beef, aged to our own specifications & perfectly seasoned. Served with hot bread & your choice of salad or cup of soup & one side-winder.

Texas 2-Step (Sizzlin' Center Cut Sirloin Platter for Two) – Two sirloin steaks served on a bed of grilled onions, topped with crispy onion strings. Served with soup or salad & a choice of one side-winder each. I ask the waitperson to ask the chef to substitute extra grilled onions for the crispy onion strings.

Smoked Sirloin – Thick slices of hickory smoked, pepper-crusted aged sirloin, slow cooked to perfection, best served medium-rare to medium.

Chopped Steak – Add sautéed mushrooms & onions for an additional charge.

Chuck's Favorite Sirloin – 7 oz. or 10 oz.

Sal's Ribeye – 10 oz. or 13 oz.

Bone-in Ribeye – "Cowboy Cut"

GR8 Center Cut Filet

Hoffbrau Filet (Bacon Wrapped) – I ask the waitperson to ask the chef to prepare my filet without the bacon.

Tenderloin Blue Cheese Salad – Thin strips of filet medallions on a bed of fresh greens , blue cheese crumbles, red onions, tomatoes, egg & bacon. I ask the waitperson to ask the chef to substitute extra tomatoes for the bacon.

Toppers:

Grilled and caramelized onion topper

Combo mushroom and onions topper

Texas sautéed mushroom topper

Chicken * Fish* Pork & More:

Served with hot bread & your choice of salad or cup of soup & one side-winder.

Grilled Chicken - Chicken breast grilled with our special house marinade.

Dr. Pepper® Chicken – Grilled chicken breast basted in Dr. Pepper® BBQ sauce, topped with mushrooms, Jack cheese & chives.

Side-Winders:

Steamed Broccoli

Steamed Spinach

Lunch Favorites:

Smaller portions of from the above menu and the following:

8 oz. New York Strip – Served with steak fries. I ask the waitperson to ask the chef to substitute steamed broccoli for the steak fries.

Grilled Chicken – Served with steamed broccoli.

Vegetable Plate – Includes the house salad and your choice of two side-winders.

Salads & Soups:

Our salad dressings are made fresh daily. Hoffbrau Steaks famous vinaigrette, creamy ranch, chunky blue cheese, and honey mustard.

Steak Salad – Top sirloin on fresh greens with bacon, egg, mixed cheese, tomato & topped with crispy onion strings. I ask the waitperson to ask the chef to substitute extra greens and tomato for the bacon and crispy onion strings.

Grilled Chicken Salad – Grilled chicken on fresh greens with bacon, egg, mixed cheese & tomato. I ask the waitperson to ask the chef to substitute extra fresh greens for the bacon.

Tenderloin Blue Cheese Salad – Thin strips of filet medallions on a bed of fresh greens, blue cheese crumbles, red onions, tomatoes, egg & bacon. I ask the waitperson to ask the chef to substitute extra red onions for the bacon.

House Salad - Fresh greens served with cheese, tomatoes & red onions (green olives upon request).

Broccoli Cheese Jalapeno Soup – Cheese soup with fresh broccoli & jalapenos.

Hoffbrau Chili

Burgers & Sandwiches:

Our burgers are 1/2 pound-fresh and are served medium-well unless requested otherwise. Served with Brau Chips. I ask the waitperson to ask the chef to substitute a vegetable for the Brau Chips.

1/2 lb. Cheeseburger – Add jalapenos or chili for an extra charge.

Honey Mustard Chicken Sandwich – Grilled chicken breast with mixed cheese, bacon, and honey mustard sauce. I ask the waitperson to ask the chef to substitute lettuce and tomato for the bacon.

Desserts:

Chocolate Chip Bread Pudding – Served with Patron XO coffee and chocolate tequila sauce.

HuHot

Mongolian Grill
Chain Restaurant

The First Conquest:

Asian Pot Stickers – Chicken and vegetable pot stickers, steamed on the grill or lightly fried. I order the grilled pot stickers.

Veggie Spring Rolls – Lightly fried and served with a sweet/spicy chili dipping sauce. I do not eat the dipping sauce.

Trusted Allies:

Soup-of-the Day (available after 4pm) – Egg Drop

Asian Salad - Greens mixed with veggies, mandarin oranges, toasted noodles and our famous Asian vinaigrette. I ask the waitperson to ask the chef to leave off the toasted noodles.

Garden Salad – Mixed greens with veggies and croutons – just enough to prepare you for battle. I ask the waitperson to ask the chef to leave off the croutons.

Chicken Salad – Mixed greens topped with your choice of breaded fried chicken or teriyaki chicken, with toasted noodles, almonds, tomatoes, mandarin oranges, broccoli, scallions, and our sweet Asian vinaigrette – a hearty meal in itself. I order the teriyaki chicken and ask the waitperson to ask the chef to leave off the toasted noodles.

The Feast: How to pillage like the Mongols. All meals are served with steamed rice.

Step 1: Prepare for battle – Advance to the fresh food bar and commandeer a bowl. Please take one bowl per trip.

Step 2: Control your destiny – Choose your favorites from a bountiful selection of meats, seafood, noodles and vegetables. Beef, chicken, mushrooms, green and red peppers, green beans, tomatoes,Spinach, broccoli, zucchini, eggs, celery, and carrots.

Step 3: Pour on the flavor. The Essential Weapon – Ladle on our specialty sauces or express your inner warrior by creating your own unique blend from the ingredients provided.

Samurai Teriyaki – a mild, slightly sweet traditional Asian favorite made with soy sauce, sugar, sherry & sesame oil.

Lemon juice, garlic oil, sesame oil, garlic broth, and ginger broth.

Not-So-Sweet-& Sour® - our version of sweet & sour; a flavorful yet mild combination of tomato sauce, vinegar, sugar & spices.

Step 4: Advance to the grill. Watch as your chosen ingredients are cooked before your eyes on our grill of epic proportions! Because I am allergic to seafood, the grill cook will clean a special section of the grill so my meal is not contaminated by seafood.

Final Pillage:

Molten Muffin – How fudge flows from this moist chocolate cake studded with chocolate chips; served warm with ice cream.

Khan's Cake – layers & layers of chocolate that's topped with more chocolate – a Genghis favorite.

Il Vincino

Wood Oven Pizza
Chain Restaurant

Pizze:

My husband and I share one regular size pizza. If I am alone, I order the small size.

<u>Pollo E Pumante</u> – Garlic oil, mozzarella, roasted chicken, sun-dried tomatoes, roasted red peppers, asiago, and fresh basil.

<u>Testarossa</u> – Marinara sauce, mozzarella, pepperoni, roasted red peppers, kalamata olives, caramelized onions, mushrooms, fresh oregano. I ask the counterperson to ask the chef to substitute extra mushrooms for the peperoni.

<u>Angeli</u> – Sweet balsamic marinara sauce, mozzarella, roasted chicken, Portobello mushrooms, artichoke hearts, gorgonzola, fresh rosemary.

Extras – for an additional charge.

Artichoke Hearts

Asiago Cheese

Kalamata Olives

Capers

Caramelized onion

Eggplant

Feta Cheese

Fontina

Fresh Tomatoes

Goat Cheese

Gorgonzola Cheese

Green Chili

Mushrooms

Pine Nuts

Red Onion

Roasted Garlic

Roasted Chicken

Roasted Red Peppers

Spinach

Sun-Dried Tomatoes

Oven Roasted Tomatoes

Pesto

Portobello Mushrooms

Turkey Sausage

Piadine: - Folded flatbread sandwiches.

Vespa – Roasted chicken, tomatoes, mayonnaise, fontina, spinach, and pesto dressing.

Tacchino – Roasted turkey, fontina, goat cheese, caramelized onions, tomatoes, romaine, and house vinaigrette.

Insalate e Zuppe:

Insalata Della Casa – Tomatoes, asiago on romaine, house vinaigrette. Add gorgonzola cheese for an additional charge.

Insalata Il Vicino – Roasted chicken, egg, tomatoes, gorgonzola, artichoke hearts, walnuts, on romaine with house dressing.

Insalata Spinaci – Gorgonzola cheese, roasted red peppers, pine nuts, red onion on fresh spinach with pesto dressing.

Zuppe Del Giorno – Soup of the Day.

Zuppa e Insalata Della Casa – Soup and salad.

Jim Bob's

Joplin, MO

Texas Size Salads:

Choice of dressing: Ranch, Bleu Cheese, Italian, French, Honey Mustard, and Raspberry Vinaigrette.

Brisket or Pulled Pork – Crisp greens and garden veggies covered in your choice of brisket or pulled pork. I always order the brisket.

Grilled Chicken Salad – Crisp mixed greens covered with grilled chicken breast, eggs, cheese, and tomatoes.

Chef's Salad – Crisp greens and garden veggies covered in turkey, ham, eggs, shredded cheese, and tomatoes. I ask the waitperson to ask the chef to give me extra turkey in place of the ham.

Homemade Chili & Soup:

Texas Chili

Soup of the day

A La Carte:

Dishes listed below are also on the side orders menu.

Creamy Cole Slaw

Sauteed Buttered Mushrooms

Fresh Veggie Medley

Dinner Salad

Steamed Broccoli

Texas Size Sandwiches:

All sandwiches are served with a generous portion of French fries. Our burgers are ½ lb. ground beef served with lettuce, tomato, pickle, and onion. On all sandwiches I ask the waitperson to ask the chef to substitute a small diner salad for the fries. On all burgers, chicken, and steak I use the bun to drain off the juices and grease then discard it.

Jim Bob Burger

Jim Bob Cheeseburger – Award-winning burger, a favorite in 4 states. With your choice of American, Jack, Swiss or cheddar cheese. I order the Swiss or cheddar cheese.

Texas Burger – With mushrooms and sour cream. I ask the waitperson to ask the chef to substitute mustard for the sour cream.

Grilled Chicken – With lettuce and tomato. Add cheese for an additional charge.

Steak Sandwich – 6oz sirloin with lettuce, tomato, and onions.

Jim Bob's Classics:

Comes with your choice of two sides and our homemade rolls. I do not eat the rolls.

Chop Steak – 12oz.

BBQ Chicken Breast

Chicken Santa Fe – Charbroiled and smothered with mushrooms, onions, tomatoes and melted cheese.

Steaks Hot off the Grill:

Hand-cut daily and marinated in herb butter makes these steaks tender and flavorful. Comes with a dinner salad, your choice of baked potato or steak fries. Oh yes! And our homemade rolls! I do not eat the rolls. I ask the waitperson to ask the chef to substitute one of the sides listed above for the potato and fries.

Texas Strip – 20 oz.

Yankee Strip – 14 oz.

<u>Bacon Wrapped Filet Mignon</u> – 9 oz. I ask the waitperson to ask the chef to leave off the bacon.

<u>Ribeye</u> – Hand-cut and grilled to perfection.

<u>Center Cut Sirloin</u> – 14 oz.

<u>Top Sirloin</u> – Award-winning 10 oz.

Kelly's Eastside

Plano, TX

Salads:

Jalapeno Ranch, Ranch, Bleu Cheese, Honey Mustard, Italian, Raspberry Vinaigrette, Balsamic Vinaigrette, or Fire Roasted Salsa dressings. All salads can be made with our House or Spinach Salad.

Dinner – Mixed greens or fresh spinach with tomato, sliced mushrooms, purple onion, cucumber and croutons. I ask the waitperson to ask the chef to substitute extra fresh spinach for the cucumber and croutons.

House – Mixed greens with tomato, grilled onions, roasted poblanos, sliced mushrooms, cheddar, hardboiled egg, cucumbers and topped with croutons. I ask the waitperson to ask the chef to substitute extra mixed greens for the cucumber and croutons.

Spinach Salad – Fresh spinach with bacon, mandarin oranges, sliced mushrooms, fire roasted almonds, grilled purple onions, roasted poblanos and topped with shredded parmesan cheese. I ask the waitperson to ask the chef to substitute extra sliced mushrooms for the bacon.

Chicken Fried Steak Salad – Fresh greens topped with our hand breaded chicken fried steak. I ask the waitperson to ask the chef to substitute grilled chicken for the chicken fried steak.

Fajita Chicken – Mouth-watering salad with grilled fajita chicken.

BBQ Salad – A special creation with our smoked brisket and sausage (regular or spicy). I ask the waitperson to ask the chef to substitute extra smoked brisket for the sausage.

Soups:

 Jailhouse Chili – Venison and beef chili topped with cheddar cheese and onions.

Burgers and Melts:

Any burger can be substituted with a grilled marinated chicken breast. All burgers are served with lettuce, tomatoes, and pickles. Your choice of one side: Coleslaw. All burgers are 1/2 pound patties.

Trio Burger – Three (1/6) patties topped with cheddar, Swiss and pepper Jack cheese.

Southwest Burger – Pepper Jack cheese, poblanos peppers, grilled red onion, guacamole, sour cream and pico de gallo top this southwestern favorite. I ask the waitperson to ask the chef to substitute extra grilled onions for the guacamole.

Plan-O-Burger – Just the usual with nothing added.

Plan-O Cheese Burger – We add lots of cheddar cheese.

Mushroom Cheese – Fresh sautéed mushrooms and Swiss cheese.

Chili Cheese – Homemade Jailhouse Chili, shredded cheddar cheese and diced onions.

The West Plano Burger – Turkey burger with guacamole, bacon and brie. I ask the waitperson to ask the chef to substitute sautéed onions for the guacamole and bacon.

Sandwiches:

All sandwiches are served with coleslaw.

BBQ Club – Sliced brisket and regular or spicy sausage with Shiner BBQ sauce and melted cheddar cheese with jalapeno ranch dressing. I ask the waitperson to ask the chef to substitute extra sliced brisket for the sausage and to leave out the middle slice of bread.

Smoked Turkey Club – Our smoked turkey with bacon,

guacamole, lettuce and tomatoes served on a hoagie roll. I ask the waitperson to ask the chef to substitute extra lettuce and tomato for the bacon and guacamole and to leave out the middle slice of bread.

Kelly's Reuben – Sliced smoked brisket and our coleslaw on three slices of grilled rye bread with pepper Jack cheese and 1000 Island dressing. I ask the waitperson to ask the chef to substitute mustard for the 1000 Island dressing and to leave out the middle slice of rye bread.

Turkey Rueben – Sliced smoked turkey and our coleslaw on three slices of grilled rye bread with Swiss cheese and 1000 Island dressing. I ask the waitperson to ask the chef to substitute mustard for the 1000 Island dressing and to leave out the middle slice of rye bread.

Sliced Beef Brisket – Smoked sliced brisket with BBQ sauce on a hoagie roll.

Grilled Hawaiian Chicken – Grilled marinated chicken breast with lettuce and tomato served on a Kaiser Roll.

Smoked Turkey and Swiss – Smoked turkey, Swiss cheese, lettuce and tomato, served on a hoagie roll.

Off the Grill:

N.Y. Strip – 12 0z. Hand cut with two sides.

Hawaiian Chicken – Marinated grilled and served on a bed of Texas rice with one side dish. I ask the waitperson to ask the chef to substitute a dinner salad or a vegetable for the rice.

Out of the Smoker:

Combination plate: choice of two or choice of three.

Sliced Beef Brisket

Half a BBQ Chicken

Grilled Beef Ribs

South of the Border:

Texas Fajitas – Marinated chicken or smoked brisket with onions, poblanos peppers, pinto beans, pico de gallo, guacamole, cheddar cheese and sour cream. I ask the waitperson to ask the chef to substitute a small salad or a vegetable for the pinto beans.

Texas Fajitas for Two – Enough fajitas and fixin's for two Texans!

Sides:

Dinner Salad

Squash & Zucchini

Vegetable de Jour

Coleslaw

Dessert:

Chocolate Pecan Pie – T.K.'s homemade warm pecan pie with chocolate chips topped with blue Bell ice cream.

Carrot Cake – The best ever layered carrot cake with cream cheese icing.

Chocolate Volcano – Hot, fresh chocolate Bundt with a scoop of Blue Bell and hot fudge topped with whipped cream and a cherry.

Skillet Cookie – Fresh baked chocolate chip cookie in its own cast iron skillet with a scoop of ice cream.

Logan's Roadhouse

Chain Restaurant

Real American Roadhouse Meals:

Craveable food at a great value every day. That's a roadhouse tradition.

Chopped Sirloin Steak 10-ounce – Smothered with Brewski Onions®, mushrooms & gravy are an extra charge. I order it without the mushrooms and gravy.

Logan's Grilled Chicken – Smothered with our own parmesan peppercorn dressing.

Teriyaki Grilled Chicken

Southwest BBQ Chicken – Smothered with BBQ sauce, Pepper Jack cheese, and tomatoes. I ask the waitperson to ask the chef to put the BBQ sauce on the side so the chicken is not smothered in it.

Premium Steakhouse Cuts:

All of our steaks are fresh, hand-cut from aged, Midwestern beef and cooked over mesquite wood. Choice of two sides. For an extra charge you can top your steak off with bleu cheese crumbles, Brewski onions ®, grilled mushrooms, sauteed mushrooms, or onions & mushroom combo

Onion Brewski® Style – We add our signature Michelob AmberBock® beer-battered onions, smothered it with garlic butter & top it off with crispy onions. I ask the waitperson to ask the chef not to put any breading on my onions and to substitute extra onions for the crispy onions.

16 oz. T-Bone – The classic cut, full of flavor.

18 oz. NY Strip – A hearty, flavorful strip steak.

12 oz. Filet Mignon – Our most tender cut of beef.

22 oz. Porterhouse – The rich flavor of a strip with the tenderness of a filet.

20 oz. Black Angus Rib Eye – Our biggest Rib Eye, well-marbled for peak flavor.

Top Sirloin Steaks:

Onion Brewski® Sirloin – Our signature 8-ounce top sirloin steak stacked on top of Michelob AmberBock® beer-braised onions, smothered with garlic butter and topped with crispy onions. I ask the waitperson to ask the chef not to put any breading on my onions and to substitute extra onions for the crispy onions.

The Logan® - Our biggest and best sirloin steak.

Sirloin – 6 oz. or 8 oz. cut.

Teriyaki Club Steak 8-ounces – Marinated in teriyaki, pineapple, herbs & spices.

Classic Cuts:

New York Strip 11-ounces

Filet Mignon 6-ounces

Logan's Filet Mignon 8-ounces

Rib-eye – 12 – ounces or 16 ounces

Logan's Prime Rib 12, 16, or 20-ounce cut

Roadhouse Combo Entrées:

Steak & Grilled Chicken – Our 6-ounce sirloin & a grilled chicken breast smothered with parmesan peppercorn dressing.

Sides & More Sides:

Brewski Onions®

House Salad

Grilled Vegetable Skewer

Grilled Mushroom Skewer

Seasonal Vegetables

Coleslaw

Caesar Salad – I ask the waitperson to ask the chef to substitute bleu cheese dressing for the Caesar dressing.

Roadies® & Burgers:

Served with home-style potato chips. I ask the waitperson to ask the chef to substitute a side for the potato chips. I do not eat the bun. I use it to drain off the juices and grease and discard it.

The Original Roadies® - Three-mini steak burgers with melted American cheese & sliced pickles on our made-from-scratch yeast rolls. I ask the waitperson to ask the chef to substitute Swiss or cheddar for the American cheese.

Roadhouse Deluxe Burger – Topped with bacon, shredded cheese, Brewski Onions ®, sauteed mushrooms, & Roadhouse BBQ sauce. I ask the waitperson to ask the chef to leave off the bacon and to put the BBQ sauce on the side.

Salads & Soups:

Kickin' Logan's Chickin' Salad – Blackened chicken over lettuce, tomatoes, cheese, & roasted corn & black bean salsa, tossed with spicy Roadhouse Ranch & crispy tortillas. I ask the waitperson to substitute extra lettuce, tomatoes and cheese for the roasted corn & black bean salsa and the crispy tortillas.

Grilled Steak Salad – Fresh Romaine & iceberg lettuce, tomatoes, shredded cheese, chopped bacon, & hard-boiled egg topped with mesquite wood-grilled steak. I ask the waitperson to ask the chef to leave off the bacon.

Anything & Everything Salad – Romaine lettuce, hard-boiled egg, bacon, bleu cheese, tomatoes, walnuts, dried cranberries, & grilled chicken with balsamic vinaigrette. I ask the waitperson to ask the chef to leave off the bacon.

Health Nuts!:

These specially prepared meals have under 550 calories. Health Nut Side Salad is Romaine lettuce, tomato & shredded carrots served with fat free vinaigrette dressing on the side. I ask the waitperson to substitute regular dressing for the fat free vinaigrette dressing. I eat these meals when I am not very hungry.

Sirloin 6-ounce cut

Mesquite Wood-Grilled Chicken

Filet Mignon 6-ounces

Health Nut Grilled Chicken Salad

"Bunless" Roadhouse Burger with a side of steamed broccoli

Mini Bucket Desserts:

Mini peanut buckets with layers of flavors. The bucket is yurs to keep!

Chocolate Brownie

Nutter Butter® Fudgeslide

Strawberry Cheesecake

Maggiano's Little Italy

Chain Restaurant

Appetizers:

Bruschetta – Fresh tomatoes, basil, balsamic vinegar & roasted garlic.

Spinach & Artichoke al Forno – Garlic crostini. I do not eat the crostini.

Tomato Caprese – Fresh Mozzarella, basil & balsamic glaze.

Soups & Salads

Can add chicken for an additional charge.

Italian Tossed Salad – Iceberg, arugula, kalamata olives, pepperoncini & Italian vinaigrette.

Caesar Salad – Grated parmesan & focaccia croutons. I ask the waitperson to ask the waiter to substitute blue cheese dressing for the Caesar dressing and to leave off the croutons.

Grilled Chicken Caprese Salad – Fresh mozzarella, tomatoes, cucumbers, kalamata olives, red onions & house dressing. I ask the waitperson to ask the chef to substitute extra tomatoes for the cucumbers.

Grilled Chicken & Apple Salad – Iceberg, arugula, grapes, celery, chives, spiced walnuts & blue cheese vinaigrette. I ask the waitperson to ask the chef to substitute extra iceberg for the grapes.

Sandwiches:

All sandwiches are served with parmesan frites. Served daily after 3 p.m. On all sandwiches I ask the waitperson to ask the chef to substitute a small dinner salad or a vegetable for the parmesan frites.

Shaved Italian Beef – Roast beef, spicy Gardiniera vegetables, mozzarella, focaccia.

Chicken Parmesan – Provolone, Marinara sauce, focaccia.

Sides:

Sautéed Spinach

Broccolini with Lemon & Garlic

Fresh Grilled Asparagus

Chicken:

Chicken Piccata – Capers & lemon butter with angel hair aglio olio. I ask the waitperson to ask the chef to substitute grilled asparagus for the angel hair aglio olio.

Chicken Marsala – Mushrooms & Marsala sauce with angel hair aglio olio. I ask the waitperson to ask the chef to substitute broccolini for the angel hair aglio olio.

Veal & Beef:

Veal Piccata - Capers & lemon butter with angel hair aglio olio. I ask the waitperson to ask the chef to substitute grilled asparagus for the angel hair aglio olio.

Veal Marsala - Mushrooms & Marsala sauce with angel hair aglio olio. I ask the waitperson to ask the chef to substitute broccolini for the angel hair aglio olio.

Veal Porterhouse – 18 oz., roasted garlic, caramelized onions & lemon with crispy red potatoes. I ask the waitperson to ask the chef to substitute sautéed spinach for the crispy red potatoes.

Beef tenderloin Medallions – Portabella & balsamic cream sauce, crispy onions & garlic mashed potatoes. I ask the waitperson to ask the chef to substitute sautéed onions for the crispy onions and broccolini for the garlic mashed potatoes.

Prime New York Steak – 16 oz. & crispy red potatoes. I ask the waitperson to ask the chef to substitute grilled asparagus for the crispy red potatoes.

<u>Center-Cut Filet Mignon</u> – 9 oz. with Italian herbs & balsamic onions with crispy red potatoes. I ask the waitperson to ask the chef to substitute broccolini for the crispy red potatoes.

Desserts:

Italian Spumoni

Seasonal Fruit

Tiramisu

Mario's Pizzeria & Ristorante

Albuquerque, NM

Appetizers:

Artichoke and Spinach Dip – A creamy hot dip of our own special recipe spinach and artichokes. Served with chips. I do not eat the chips.

Soup & Salad:

Antipasto Salad - A deluxe Italian salad with Genoa salami, artichoke hearts, ham, provolone, tomatoes, black and green olives and pepperoncini on a mound of mixed greens. I ask the waitperson to ask the chef to substitute extra tomatoes for the ham.

Greek Salad – Feta cheese, kalamata olives, cucumbers, artichoke hearts, pepperoncini and red onions. Served on a bed of mixed greens with Greek herb dressing.

Mario's Chopped Salad – Cappiola ham, Genoa salami, feta, cheddar and mozzarella cheeses, black and green olives, red onions, cucumbers and tomatoes atop a bed of freshly chopped lettuce. Tossed in our own house vinaigrette. I ask the waitperson to ask the chef to substitute extra tomatoes and chopped lettuce for the ham and cucumbers.

Chicken Caesar Salad – Grilled chicken, tomatoes, croutons, parmigiano and Romano cheeses tossed with romaine and creamy Caesar dressing. I ask the waitperson to ask the chef to substitute extra tomatoes for the croutons and to substitute blue cheese dressing for the Caesar dressing.

Cobb Salad – Turkey, ham, Genoa salami, provolone, cheddar, mozzarella, bacon, eggs and tomatoes served on a bed of mixed greens. I ask the waitperson to ask the chef to substitute extra turkey for the ham and bacon.

Sante Fe Chicken Salad – Grilled Chicken, cheddar and mozzarella cheeses, green chili, sunflower seeds, red onions, tomatoes and tortilla chips on a bed of mixed greens, I ask the waitperson to ask the chef to substitute extra red onions for the tortilla chips.

Soup and Salad – Homemade soup, garden salad and our homemade bread sticks.

Homemade Soups – Minestrone or soup of the day.

Dressing Selections:

House Italian

Buttermilk Ranch

Bleu Cheese

Honey Mustard

Chicken:

Served with your choice of homemade soup or fresh garden salad and garlic bread. A low carb substitution of steamed vegetables can be had in place of pasta for an additional charge.

Southwest Chicken – Grilled chicken, mushroom and diced tomatoes tossed with penne pasta in our green chili alfredo. I order this dish with steamed vegetables in place of the penne pasta.

Chicken Marsala – Chicken breast sautéed in Marsala cream sauce with fresh mushrooms and onions. Served with a side of spaghetti. I order this dish with the steamed vegetables in place of the spaghetti.

Chicken Cacciatore – Chicken breast sautéed in white wine marinara, bell peppers, onions, mushrooms, and olives. Served with a side of spaghetti. I order this dish with the steamed vegetables in place of the spaghetti.

Chicken Piccata – Chicken breast, capers, onions and mushrooms sautéed in olive oil, white wine and lemons. Served with a side of spaghetti. I order this dish with steamed vegetables in place of spaghetti.

Italian Subs:

Served with coleslaw. Add a cup of soup or a dinner salad to any sub for an additional charge. Add sautéed bell peppers and onions for an additional charge.

Meatball Parmigianino Sub – Mama's homemade meatballs smothered in meat sauce, Romano and mozzarella cheese.

Italian Cheese Steak Sub – Grilled roast beef, sautéed onions, bell jpeppers, mushrooms and melted provolone.

Sandwiches:

Served with coleslaw. Add a cup of soup or a dinner salad to any sub for an additional charge. Add sautéed bell peppers and onions for an additional charge.

Uptown Turkey – Sliced breast of turkey, green chili, melted provolone cheese, lettuce, tomatoes and mayo.

New York Reuben – Triple decker hot pastrami, sliced turkey, sauerkraut, mustard and provolone cheese. Served on grilled rye. I ask the waitperson to ask the chef serve this sandwich both open faced and without the middle slice of bread.

French Dip – Lean roast beef topped with provolone, served with au jus.

Hot Pastrami – Thinly sliced lean pastrami, provolone, mustard, lettuce, tomatoes on grilled rye.

Mario's Stack – Your choice of roast beef or grilled chicken breast. Topped with green chili, melted cheddar cheese, lettuce, tomatoes, mayo and Italian dressing.

Pizza Burger – Smothered with marinara sauce and mozzarella cheese.

Philly Burger – Sautéed peppers, onions and provolone cheese.

Green Chile Cheeseburger

Mimi's Café

Enjoy a Taste of France
Chain Restaurant

Starters & Small Plates:

Petite Wedge – Crisp iceberg lettuce topped with bacon, diced tomatoes, red onions and bleu cheese crumbles. Served with your choice of dressing. I ask the waitperson to substitute extra diced tomatoes for the bacon.

Spinach & Artichoke Dip – Creamy dip with sundried tomatoes and four cheeses. Served with a grilled garlic sourdough baguette. I do not eat the baguette.

Signature Soups:

French Onion – A traditional favorite with Swiss, mozzarella, and parmesan cheeses. I ask the waitperson to ask the chef to leave off the bread and croutons.

Soup du Jour – Ask about our soup of the day.

Café Salads:

Add a cup of soup for an extra charge. Chicken can be added for an extra charge.

Bleu Cheese & Walnut – Baby greens, dried cranberries, bacon, tomatoes, and strawberries tossed in balsamic vinaigrette. I order the chicken and ask the waitperson to ask the chef to substitute extra tomatoes for the bacon.

Mediterranean Salad – Baby greens, feta cheese, tomatoes, pistachios, and dried cranberries tossed in balsamic vinaigrette. I order the chicken.

Mimi's Chopped Cobb – Turkey, bacon avocado, green onions, egg, tomatoes, and crumbled bleu cheese. I ask the waitperson to ask the chef to substitute extra tomatoes and green onions for the bacon and avocado.

Asian Chopped - Roasted chicken breast, cabbage, Romaine, carrots, cilantro, wontons, green onions, red & green peppers, and sesame dressing. I ask the waitperson to ask the chef to substitute extra Romaine for the wontons.

Artisan Sandwiches & Bistro Burgers:

Includes your choice of coleslaw. Substitute a cup of homemade soup or fresh fruit for an extra charge.

Fresh Roasted Turkey Club – Bacon, lettuce, tomato and mayonnaise on toasted sourdough. I ask the waitperson to ask the chef to substitute extra lettuce and tomato for the bacon.

Classic Beef Dip – Thinly sliced top round roast served on a grilled sourdough baguette. For an extra charge add cheese, grilled onions, peppers, and mushrooms.

Our Bistro Burgers are made with 100% ground chuck. A turkey patty is available upon request.

French Quarter - Avocado, bacon, Swiss cheese and 1000 island on grilled parmesan sourdough. Served with lettuce, tomato, onions, and pickles. I ask the waitperson to ask the chef to substitute extra tomato and onions for the avocado and the bacon.

Classic Burger – Lettuce, tomato, onions, and pickles.

Mimi's Cheeseburger – Your choice of cheese, lettuce, tomato, onions, and pickles.

Café Classics:

Add a soup or a garden salad for an extra charge.

Slow Roasted Turkey Breast – Homemade mashed potatoes, gravy, cornbread dressing, fresh vegetables, and orange cranberry relish. I ask the waitperson to ask the chef to substitute a garden salad for the mashed potatoes, gravy, and cornbread dressing.

Oven Fresh Pot Roast – Slowly braised chuck roast with

mashed potatoes, gravy, and fresh vegetables. I ask the waitperson to ask the chef to substitute a garden fresh salad for the mashed potatoes and gravy.

Grilled Meatloaf – House-made and slow cooked. Served with mashed potatoes, gravy, and fresh vegetables. I ask the waitperson to ask the chef to substitute a garden fresh salad for the mashed potatoes and gravy.

Pasta:

For an extra charge add a soup or a garden salad.

Mediterranean Fettuccini – Tossed with spinach, sundried tomatoes, artichoke hearts and tomato Asiago cream sauce. Topped with fresh diced tomatoes and grated parmesan cheese. Add chicken for an additional charge. I order the chicken.

Gourmet François:

Cheddar & Broccoli Quiche – Served with baby greens, fresh fruit, and a freshly baked muffin. I do not eat the muffin.

Turkey Pistachio Salad Croissant – Turkey, pistachios and dried cranberries blended with mayonnaise and Dijon mustard with lettuce and tomato. Served with coleslaw.

Fresh & Fit:

All Mimi's Café Fresh & Fit items are 550 calories or less. I do not eat these dishes because they are low in calories. I eat them because they taste good.

Broiled Chicken & Fruit Plate – Chicken breast with baby spring greens, tomatoes, and fresh seasonal fruit.

Petite Filet – Broiled center cut beef tenderloin, vegetables and balsamic baby greens.

Slow Roasted Turkey Breast – With orange cranberry relish, brown rice and fresh steamed vegetables. I ask the waitperson to ask the chef to substitute extra fresh steamed vegetables for the rice.

Desserts:

Mimi's Bread Pudding - baked from scratch with plump raisins, vanilla and special spice blend. Served warm with buttery whiskey sauce.

Fresh Apple Cinnamon Crisp – Topped with golden buttery crumbles and served warm with vanilla bean ice cream.

Triple Chocolate Brownie – Served warm with vanilla bean ice cream and topped with chocolate and caramel sauces.

Montana Mike's Steakhouse

Chain Restaurant

Starters:

Spinach and Artichoke Dip – Melted parmesan and mozzarella cheeses blended with spinach and artichoke, accompanied by diced tomatoes. Served with tri-colored fried tortilla chips. I do not eat the tortilla chips.

Salads:

Buffalo Chicken Salad – Buffalo-style tenders blended with peppered bacon, pepper Jack cheese, tortilla straws, candied pecans, tomatoes, red onion and bell peppers. Served on a bed of greens and tossed with garlic ranch dressing. (Substitute grilled chicken or breaded tender strips.) I order the grilled chicken and ask the waitperson to ask the chef to substitute extra tomatoes for the bacon and tortilla straws.

Chicken Tostada Salad – Grilled chicken with shredded cheese, peppered bacon and tortilla strips. Served with chipotle ranch dressing. I ask the waitperson to ask the chef to substitute extra greens for the bacon and tortilla strips.

Open Range Chicken Caesar Salad - Grilled chicken on a bed of crisp romaine lettuce, garlic croutons, parmesan cheese and classic Caesar dressing. I ask the waitperson to ask the chef to substitute extra romaine lettuce for the croutons and to substitute bleu cheese dressing for the Caesar dressing.

Mike's Garden Fresh House Salad – A pile of greens with croutons, tomatoes, shredded cheese, onions, and bacon bits. Add chicken breast or grilled Angus Sirloin Steak for an additional charge. I ask the waitperson to ask the chef to substitute extra tomatoes for the croutons and bacon bits.

Steaks:

All entrées include our garden salad with your choice of

dressing, one Mike's side, and a freshly-baked roll.

<u>Center Cut Top Sirloin Steaks</u> – Our sirloin steaks are naturally aged and grilled over an open flame. 6oz., 8oz., or 11oz.

<u>Ancho Pepper Crusted Sirloin</u> – Our 11oz. center-cut sirloin seasoned with ancho pepper and topped with ancho butter.

<u>Mike's Big Montana Steak</u> – A 22oz. sirloin sure to satisfy mountain-size appetite.

<u>Kansas City Strip</u> – The cattleman's favorite cut.

<u>Filet Mignon</u> – Applewood bacon-wrapped tenderloin filet seasoned, grilled, and lightly brushed with butter. You won't get a more tender cut than this! 8oz. or 12oz. I ask the waitperson to ask the chef to leave off the bacon.

<u>Ribeye Steak</u> – Tender, juicy and flavorful. Mountain Momma Ribeye – 12 oz. Mile High Ribeye – 16 oz.

<u>The "44" Sirloin</u> – Perfect for two, unless you want to go it alone. Comes with two setups to complete the deal.

<u>Porterhouse</u> – The king of Steaks! A 24 oz. strip and filet in one thick cut that will satisfy any appetite.

<u>Rancher's T-Bone</u> – A full pound of flavor that's good to the bone.

<u>Buffalo Steak</u> – With creamy peppercorn sauce ....Buffalo has the juicy taste of beef and has less fat than a boneless, skinless chicken breast.

<u>Prime Rib</u> – (Served 4pm to close Friday & Saturday, while it lasts.) Mike's aged prime rib is seasoned, seared and slow-roasted. Hand carved to order and served with traditional au jus. Regular cut or Mikes cut.

Mike's Sides:

Sautéed Button Mushrooms

Steamed Veggies

Green Beans

Garden Salad

Cole Slaw

Open Range Caesar Salad – see above.

Sautéed Sliced Mushrooms

Other favorites:

Mountain Topper - Chopped sirloin or flame-grilled chicken topped with bacon, sautéed mushrooms, shredded Jack/cheddar cheese and a touch of honey mustard. I ask the waitperson to ask the chef to substitute extra mushrooms for the bacon.

Mike's Angus Kebobs – Tender pieces of marinated sirloin, grilled with onions, red peppers and green peppers.

Teriyaki Glazed Chicken – Chicken breast flame-grilled with teriyaki glaze, sesame seeds and grilled pineapple over a bed of rice. I ask the waitperson to substitute extra pineapple for the rice.

Flame Grilled Chicken Breast

Chopped Angus Sirloin Steak – with mushroom gravy. I ask the waitperson to ask the chef to substitute grilled or sautéed mushrooms for the mushroom gravy.

Sirloin Angus Beef Tips – Served on a bed of rice with grilled onions, peppers, and mushroom gravy. I ask the waitperson to ask the chef to substitute extra grilled onions for the rice and mushroom gravy.

Great Combos:

Angus Steak & Chicken – Sirloin steak with a grilled chicken breast.

Burgers:

Served with our toasted bun with Mike's fries. All of Mike's burgers are made from a ½ pound of fresh ground Angus beef. I ask the waitperson to ask the chef to substitute broccoli or green beans for the fries.

The Mountain Burger - A one pound burger! Served with lettuce, tomato, pickle and onion. Your choice of mustard or mayo.

Buffalo Burger – Lean, flavorful and all-natural bison topped with melted Jack/cheddar cheese, pickle, our homemade hickory sauce and 2 fried onion rings. I ask the waitperson to ask the chef to leave off the hickory sauce and to substitute extra broccoli for the onion rings.

Hamburger – Served with lettuce, tomato, pickle, and onion. Your choice of mustard or mayo.

Bacon Swiss Mushroom Burger – Served with Applewood bacon, Swiss cheese, sautéed mushrooms, mayonnaise, lettuce, pickle, tomato and onion. I ask the waitperson to ask the chef to substitute extra tomato for the bacon.

Roadhouse Grilled Chicken – Served with sautéed onions and peppers, honey mustard and Swiss cheese on a Ciabatta bun.

Grilled Chicken Breast – Served with lettuce, pickle, tomato, onion and mayo on a Ciabatta bun.

Lunch Features:

Lunch Served Monday – Friday 11 am – 4pm. All entrées include a salad, freshly baked roll, and choice of side. Features are the same meals that listed above but are served in lunch size portions.

Noshville Delicatessen

Nashville, TN

Egg Dishes:

Served with choice of silver $ potato cakes, fresh fruit, oatmeal, sliced tomatoes, toast, or bagel. I order all my eggs with sliced tomatoes.

Egg Dishes:

2 Eggs Any Style

Eggs and Onions

Omelets:

Spinach & Cheese Omelet

Vegetable Omelet

Western Omelet – I ask the waitperson to ask the chef to leave out the ham.

Create Your Own Omelet

Spicy Chicken & Pepper Jack Cheese Omelet

Tomato & Cheese Omelet

Check This Out!:

Potato Pancakes – I eat potato pancakes on a reward day.

Cheese Blintzes

Homemade Soups;

Sweet & Sour Cabbage

Vegetable Soup

Fresh Salads:

Greek Salad

Chicken Curry Salad

Cobb Salad – I ask the waitperson to ask the chef to leave off the ham.

Spinach Salad

Tossed salad

Delicatessen Sandwiches:

Served with Coleslaw. I order all sandwiches open faced.

Fresh Roasted Turkey

Turkey Pastrami

Pastrami

Corned Beef

Rare Roast Beef

Brisket

O'Charley's

Chain Restaurant

Appetizers:

<u>Authentic Spinach & Artichoke Dip</u> – A warm creamy blend of spinach and artichoke hearts sprinkled with parmesan cheese. Served warm with crisp tortilla chips. I do not eat the tortilla chips.

Signature Salads:

<u>Pecan Chicken Tender Salad</u> – Pecan-crusted chicken tossed with mandarin oranges, dried cranberries, bleu cheese crumbles and candied pecans. Served with our balsamic vinaigrette.

<u>California Chicken Salad</u> – Grilled chicken, bleu cheese crumbles, candied pecans, fresh ripe strawberries, mandarin oranges and dried cranberries tossed in a romaine and spring mix and served with our balsamic vinaigrette.

<u>Calypso Spinach Salad</u> – Grilled chicken, thinly sliced and tossed with fresh baby spinach, green apples, bacon, dried cranberries, candied pecans, bleu cheese crumbles, and thinly sliced red onions. All tossed with our honey-apple cider vinaigrette. I ask the waitperson to ask the chef to substitute extra spinach for the bacon.

<u>Black & Bleu Caesar Salad</u> – Blackened, grilled USDA choice sirloin and crumbled bleu cheese on top of crisp romaine lettuce, fresh tomatoes and bacon. Tossed with our Caesar dressing. I ask the waitperson to ask the chef to substitute extra tomatoes for the bacon and to substitute bleu cheese dressing for the Caesar dressing.

Salad Dressings:

Honey Mustard

Oil & Vinegar

Balsamic Vinaigrette

Honey-Apple Cider Vinaigrette

Ranch

Bleu Cheese

Side Items:

Soup

Salad

Broccoli

Broccoli Cheese Casserole

Fresh Asparagus

Pasta:

Prime Rib Pasta – Tender prime rib, Applewood-smoked bacon, asparagus and mushrooms tossed with penne pasta and our Sun-Dried Tomato Alfredo sauce, and then finished with a Cajun-Horseradish sauce. I ask the waitperson to ask the chef to substitute extra mushrooms for the bacon.

Cajun Chicken Pasta – Grilled chicken, peppers, onions and parmesan cheese tossed with linguini in our spicy New Orleans cream sauce.

Chicken Italia – Grilled chicken breast with mozzarella, tomatoes, asparagus and lemon butter. Served atop linguini tossed with parmesan cheese and garlic butter.

Teriyaki Sesame Chicken – Thinly sliced grilled chicken breast basted with teriyaki sauce and tossed with garlic, red pepper flakes, Sesame-Pineapple sauce, mushrooms, peppers and onions. Served on a bed of rice pilaf. I ask the waitperson to ask the chef to substitute extra peppers and onions for the rice.

Butcher's Cut Premium Steaks:

All steaks are served with a choice of two side items.

Louisiana Sirloin – Our signature 12 oz. sirloin is rubbed with a secret blend of Cajun seasonings, cooked to perfection and topped with Cajun butter.

Grilled Top Sirloin – Our juicy USDA Choice sirloin, perfectly seasoned and cooked just the way you like it. 6 oz., 9 oz., or 12 oz.

Your Favorite Rib-Eye Steak – For the serious steak lover, a hearty 12 oz. cut, generously marbled and seasoned for maximum flavor, then grilled to order.

Prime Time Prim Rib – Hand-rubbed with herbs and spices, slow-roasted in our very own kitchen, then sliced to order. Available Friday after 4:00pm and all day Saturday and Sunday while it lasts. 12 oz. cut or 16 oz. cut.

Filet Mignon – We patiently age 8 thick ounces of beef to give you our most tender, mouthwatering steak. Seasoned and grilled to order.

1/2 lb. Burgers:

All burgers are cooked to order and served with hot, seasoned fries. I ask the waitperson to ask the chef to substitute one of the side items for the fries.

Classic Burger A juicy 100% all-beef burger topped with lettuce, tomato, onion and pickles. Cheddar cheese is an extra charge.

Grilled Turkey Burger – A seasoned all-white meat turkey patty topped with melted Jack cheese and your favorite toppings. Served with your choice of side item.

Sandwiches:

Philly Cheese Steak – Thinly sliced slow-roasted prime rib piled on a toasted roll and topped with sautéed mushrooms, peppers and spicy queso

Desserts:

Brownie Lover's Brownie – Our decadent chocolate brownie filled with toffee morsels, and drizzled with chocolate and caramel sauces, then topped with Blue Bell® Vanilla Bean ice cream.

Olive Garden

Chain Restaurant

With any entrée, enjoy garden-fresh salad prepared just for you, or one of our delicious soups made from scratch. Served with freshly baked garlic breadsticks. I always chose the salad and do not eat the breadsticks.

We will gladly substitute whole wheat linguine for any pasta or vegetables for any side.

Antipasti (Appetizers):

Hot Artichoke-Spinach Dip – A blend of artichokes, spinach and cream cheese. Served with Tuscan bread. I do not eat the bread.

Smoked Mozzarella Fonduta – Oven-baked smoked mozzarella, provolone, parmesan, and Romano cheese. Served with Tuscan bread. I do not eat the bread.

Zuppe e Insalate (Soups & Salads):

Grilled Chicken Caesar Salad – Grilled chicken over romaine in a creamy Caesar dressing topped with parmesan cheese and croutons. I ask the wait person to ask the chef to leave off the croutons and to substitute Italian dressing for the Caesar dressing.

Garden-Fresh Salad – Our famous house salad, tossed with our signature Italian dressing.

Cucina Classica (Classic Recipes):

I eat these classic recipe dishes on reward nights.

Spaghetti with Meat Sauce – Traditional meat sauce seasoned with garlic and herbs over spaghetti. Meatballs are an extra charge.

Chicken Parmigiana – Parmesan-breaded chicken breasts fried and topped with marinara sauce and mozzarella cheese. Served with spaghetti. I ask the waitperson to ask the chef to substitute broccoli for the spaghetti.

Eggplant Parmigiana – Lightly breaded eggplant fried and topped with marinara sauce mozzarella, and parmesan cheese. Served with spaghetti. I ask the waitperson to ask the chef to substitute broccoli for the spaghetti.

Lighter Italian Fare:

Flavorful Entrées Under 575 Calories. I do not eat these dishes because they are low in calories. I eat them because they taste good.

Venetian Apricot Chicken. – Grilled chicken breasts in an apricot citrus sauce. Served with broccoli, asparagus, and diced tomatoes.

Pollo (Chicken):

Moscato Peach Chicken – Grilled chicken breasts with a moscato wine and peach glaze served with spinach, tomatoes, and curly mafada pasta in a creamy parmesan sauce with as touch of pancetta bacon. I ask the waitperson to ask the chef to leave off the pancetta bacon. On non-reward days I ask to have broccoli substituted for the mafada pasta.

Stuffed Chicken Marsala – Oven-roasted chicken breasts stuffed with Italian cheeses and sun-dried tomatoes, topped with mushrooms and a creamy marsala sauce with a touch of pancetta bacon. I ask the waitperson to ask the chef to leave off the pancetta bacon.

Carne (Beef & Pork):

Mixed Grill – Skewers of grilled marinated steak and chicken with a rosemary demi-glace, served with grilled vegetables and Tuscan potatoes. I ask the waitperson to ask the chef to substitute extra grilled vegetables for the potatoes.

Steak Toscano – Grilled 12 oz. choice center cut strip steak brushed with Italian herbs and extra-virgin olive oil. Served with Tuscan potatoes and bell peppers. I ask the wait person to ask the chef to substitute either grilled vegetables or broccoli for the potatoes.

Lunch Entrées:

The same meals in smaller portions are available for lunch.

Dolci (Desserts):

Tiramisu – The classic Italian dessert. A layer of creamy custard set atop espresso-soaked ladyfingers.

White Chocolate Raspberry Cheesecake – Raspberry-swirled white chocolate cheese cake topped with slivers of white chocolate.

Dolcini – Piccoli Dolci "little dessert treats", layered with cake, pastry creams, and berries. Strawberry & White Chocolate, Amaretto Tiramisu, and Dark Chocolate Caramel Cream.

Rafferty's Restaurant & Bar

Chain Restaurant

Soups & Crisp Fresh Salads:

Rafferty's Lunch Duos – Daily from 11:00AM – 4:00PM. Choose any two. Bowl of Soup/House Salad/1/2 Club Sandwich/Caesar Salad/Bowl of Fruit.

Soup of the Day – Ask your server for today's fresh-made soup.

House Salad – Fresh crisp mixed greens with chopped eggs, diced tomatoes, crisp potato sticks and hot chopped bacon. Topped with your choice of dressing. I ask the waitperson to ask the chef to substitute extra mixed greens and tomatoes for the potato sticks and bacon.

House Salad & Soup – A great combination! Our piping hot made-from-scratch soup and crisp fresh house salad topped with your choice of dressing.

Chicken Finger Salad – A Rafferty's classic! Cold mixed greens topped with chopped eggs, fresh diced tomatoes, crispy potato sticks, Monterey Jack cheese, and chopped fried chicken finger filets. I ask the waitperson to ask the chef to substitute extra mixed greens for the potato sticks and to substitute grilled chicken for the fried chicken finger filets.

The Chef – Fresh greens topped with smoked turkey, ham, Monterey Jack and cheddar cheeses, chopped eggs, fresh diced tomatoes, crisp potato sticks and hot chopped bacon. I ask the waitperson to ask the chef to substitute extra turkey for the ham and bacon and to substitute extra fresh greens for the potato sticks.

Caesar Salad – Fresh hearts of romaine lettuce tossed to order with seasoned croutons, Parmesan cheese and Caesar dressing. Add grilled chicken for an additional charge. I ask the waitperson to ask the chef to substitute extra romaine lettuce for the croutons and to substitute bleu cheese dressing for the Caesar dressing.

Frisco Salad – Seasoned grilled chicken, chopped eggs, fresh diced tomatoes, crispy potato sticks, Monterey Jack cheese and artichoke hearts on a bed of cool crisp greens. Topped with Rafferty's own vinaigrette dressing. I ask the waitperson to ask the chef to substitute extra diced tomatoes for the potato sticks.

Rafferty's Homemade Chicken Salad:

Sunshine Chicken Salad – Our homemade chicken salad served with fresh fruit and melons. Topped with chopped mixed nuts and sweet orange dressing. A lunchtime favorite! I ask the waitperson to ask the chef to substitute tomatoes for the melons.

Chicken Salad, Croissants & Soup – Two croissants served with Rafferty's homemade chicken salad and choice of soup. I eat the croissants on a reward day.

Dressings:

House Honey-Mustard

Garlic Ranch

Bleu Cheese

Vinaigrette

Chicken:

Chicken entrées served with one side item. Add a salad for an additional charge.

Kona Chicken – A boneless chicken breast marinated in pineapple juice and soy sauce grilled over hickory wood then topped with grilled ham, Monterey Jack cheese and a slice of pineapple. I ask the waitperson to ask the chef to substitute extra Monterey Jack cheese for the ham.

BBQ Chicken – Hickory-grilled chicken breast basted with our sweet & zesty BBQ sauce then topped with Monterey Jack cheese and hickory smoked bacon. I ask the waitperson to ask the chef to substitute extra Monterey Jack cheese for the smoked bacon.

Sandwiches:

Bluegrass Special – A boneless marinated hickory-grilled BBQ chicken breast topped with bacon, Monterey Jack cheese, pickles, sliced tomatoes, lettuce and mayonnaise. Served on your choice of toasted egg bun or toasted wheatberry bread. I ask the waitperson to ask the chef to substitute extra tomatoes for the bacon.

French Dip – Thinly shaved prime rib smothered with melted Monterey Jack. Served on French loaf, au jus.

Open-Faced Prime Rib Sandwich – (available after 4:00PM) A juicy cut of our slow-roasted prime rib served on French loaf. Served au jus.

1/2 lb. Black Angus Burgers:

Rafferty's American Cheeseburger – A thick juicy Black Angus chuck patty grilled on hickory wood then topped with American cheese, crisp lettuce, sliced tomatoes, onions, pickles, mayo and mustard. Served on a toasted egg bun. I ask the waitperson to ask the chef to substitute Monterey Jack cheese for the American cheese.

Backyard BBQ Burger – A Black Angus chuck patty topped with smoked bacon, charcoal grilled sweet onions, smoked cheddar cheese and BBQ sauce. I ask the waitperson to ask the chef to substitute extra grilled sweet onions for the smoked bacon.

Sides:

Creamy Cole Slaw

Broccoli

Fresh Fruit Bowl

Steaks & Chops:

Choose from these three savory toppings: Hickory grilled & lightly seasoned for that classic Rafferty's flavor; Six Shooter

Cajun Butter rubbed with a zingy blend of six herbs and spices; Bleu Cheese Butter made with fresh bleu cheese crumbles.

Cowboy Sirloin – A tender, juicy 10 oz. sirloin.

Ribeye – A hearty 12 oz. Ribeye steak well-marbled for full-bodied taste.

Rafferty's Specialty Beef:

Served with one side item. Add a salad for an additional charge.

Slow-Roasted Prime Rib – (available after 4:00pm) Our aged USDA choice prime rib is seasoned then slow-roasted for tenderness and flavor. Hand-carved to order and served au jus.

Jackson Hole Filet – A thick & juicy 8 oz. filet slow-roasted over hickory wood. The most tender of all our steaks.

Classic Marinated Ribeye – A 12 oz. Ribeye marinated in pineapple juice & soy sauce for a great savory taste.

BBQ Ribs & Combos:

Sirloin Steak & Chicken Finger Combo – A 10 oz. sirloin grilled just the way you like it paired with five chicken finger filets. I ask the waitperson to ask the chef to substitute grilled chicken for the chicken finger filets.

Desserts:

The Brookie – A tasty combination of a coconut chocolate nut brownie and a cookie. Crowned with rich French vanilla ice cream, drizzled with Hershey's chocolate syrup.

Range Café

Albuquerque & Bernalillo, NM

Appetizers:

Creamy Spinach Artichoke Dip – Parmesan, white cheddar, cream cheese with garlic toast, salsa.

Soups:

Homemade Soup of the Day – Served with fresh bread.

Green Chile Chicken Stew – It's a soup that eats like a meal, served with a flour tortilla on the side. Chicken, carrots, potatoes, peas, green beans, and chilies.

Salads:

Dressings: Raspberry Vinaigrette, Bleu Cheese, Balsamic Vinaigrette, Ranch, Sun-Dried Tomato Vinaigrette, and Dijon Vinaigrette.

Range Wedge – Crisp iceberg, Gorgonzola, chopped bacon, tomato, balsamic vinaigrette, ranch dressing. I ask the waitperson to ask the chef to substitute extra tomatoes for the bacon.

Caesar – Romaine, homemade croutons, parmesan, classic Caesar dressing. Add chilled seasoned chicken for an additional charge. I ask the waitperson to ask the chef to substitute bleu cheese dressing for the Caesar dressing and to leave off the croutons.

Cobb – Romaine, turkey breast, avocado, bacon, boiled egg, tomato, red onions, and Gorgonzola. I ask the waitperson to ask the chef to substitute extra tomato and red onions for the avocado and bacon.

Chicken Salad Chef – House-made chicken salad, crisp iceberg, romaine, tomato, fresh asparagus, cucumber, red onion, boiled egg, and white cheddar. I ask the waitperson to ask the chef to substitute extra tomato for the cucumber.

Rio Rojo – Romaine, artichoke hearts, tomato, Gorgonzola cheese, red onion, balsamic vinaigrette. Add chilled seasoned chicken or grilled N.Y. steak for an additional charge.

Burgers:

Our all natural fresh Angus burgers are 8 oz. flame grilled to order, served on a fresh bun with lettuce, tomato, onion, pickle, choice of house salad or Range slaw.

Range Original – Build it however you please.

Bernalillo – Bacon, green chili, and white cheddar cheese. I ask the waitperson to ask the chef to substitute extra tomato for the bacon.

Wyoming – Sautéed mushrooms, grilled onion, and Swiss cheese.

Ponderosa – Bleu cheese, topped with onion rings. I ask the waitperson to ask the chef to substitute grilled onions for the onion rings.

Relleno – Topped with a blue corn chili relleno, green chili sauce and white cheddar cheese.

Sandwiches:

Served with a choice of house salad or Range slaw.

Camino Del Pueblo – Grilled chicken breast, bleu cheese, sautéed mushrooms, topped with onion rings, Dijon mayo on a fresh bun. I ask the waitperson to ask the chef to substitute grilled onions for the onion rings.

Meatloaf Sandwich – Tom's recipe, lettuce, tomato, mayo, and a hoagie roll.

Chicken Salad – Poached chicken breast, diced veggies, mayo, served open-faced on cinnamon raisin bread.

Range Favorites:

Tom's Meatloaf – A Range favorite since day one! Range mashed potatoes, mushroom gravy, and fresh veggies. I ask the waitperson to ask the chef to substitute extra fresh veggies for the mashed potatoes.

Hot Turkey Plate – Roasted turkey breast, stuffing, Range mashed potatoes, green chili gravy, and fresh veggies. I ask the waitperson to ask the chef to substitute a dinner salad and extra fresh veggies for the stuffing and mashed potatoes.

Rio Grande Gorge – 8 oz. ground chuck beef patty served open-faced on a tortilla, topped with red or green chili sauce, white cheddar, grilled onions, Range fries con queso, and black beans. I ask the waitperson to ask the chef to substitute fresh veggies and a dinner salad for the Range fries con queso and black beans.

Dinner:

Served after 4pm, includes all lunch items. Add a side soup or a mixed green salad for an additional charge.

Range Supper Favorites:

El Sueno De Vaquero – 10 oz. grilled New York Strip topped with chipotle compound butter, topped with onion rings, served with Range mashed potatoes, and fresh asparagus. I ask the waitperson to ask the chef to substitute grilled onions for the onion rings and fresh veggies for the mashed potatoes.

Rosemary Penne Pasta – Fresh herbs, artichoke hearts, sun-dried tomatoes, fresh spinach and creamy Parmesan sauce over penne pasta. Add grilled chicken for an additional charge. I eat the pasta on a reward night.

Range Chicken – Grilled chicken breast, white corn tortillas, chili con queso, chopped green chili, melted white cheddar, topped with sliced avocado, and served with black beans and arroz verde. I ask the waitperson to ask the chef to substitute fresh vegetables and a dinner salad for the avocado, black beans, and arroz verde.

Desserts:

Life by Chocolate – Premium Callebaut Belgian white chocolate, raspberry-white chocolate, mocha milk chocolate and dark chocolate mousses layered together and glazed with rich ganache.

Amaretto Bread Pudding – With raisins, toasted almonds, served warm with Amaretto butter sauce.

Chocolate Roadhouse Cake – Moist, rich chocolate cake layered with thick chocolate fudge frosting.

Crème Brulee – Baked Vanilla bean custard topped with caramelized sugar.

Brownie Sundae – Warm walnut fudge brownie topped with your choice of premium ice cream and caramel sauce.

Chocolate Pinon Torte – A decadent nearly flourless chocolate torte with toasted pinon nuts, a hint of cinnamon finished with dark chocolate shavings and chocolate ganache.

Rib Crib

Chain Restaurant

Fresh Salads:

Smoked Chicken Caesar Salad – Marinated chicken, smoked, then sliced and served on salad greens with a topping of Parmesan cheese and creamy Caesar dressing. I ask the wait person to ask the chef to substitute blue cheese dressing for the Caesar dressing.

Smoked Chicken Salad – A salad and then some. Tender, juicy, slow-smoked chicken on fresh greens with tomatoes, shredded cheese, and crispy tortilla strips. I order blue cheese dressing and ask the waitperson to ask the chef to leave off the tortilla strips.

Dynamite Chicken Salad – This salad packs some serious POW! Succulent slices of hickory-smoked chicken breast add savory flavor to a salad of fresh greens, Southwest corn medley, tomatoes and cheese. Garnished with three cheese quesadilla roll-ups and served with BBQ ranch dressing. I ask the waitperson to ask the chef to give me the cheese but to leave off the quesadillas.

Fire-Grilled Burgers:

On all burgers, I do not eat the bun. I use it to drain off the juices then I discard it.

The Crib Fire ® Burger – This bad boy is built! We start with an onion ring, add a seasoned, all-beef patty, then pile on a spicy hot link, pepper jack and cheddar cheeses and a dash of mild BBQ sauce. With a side of seasoned fries. I ask the waitperson to ask the chef to substitute raw onion for the onion ring, leave off the spicy hot link, and to substitute a small salad for the fries.

BBQ Bacon Cheeseburger – Thick-cut peppered bacon and caramelized onions add a swift kick of flavor to a seasoned beef patty that's fire-grilled and finished with BBQ sauce, cheddar cheese, fresh lettuce and tomato. With a side of seasoned fries. I ask the waitperson to ask the chef to leave off the bacon and to substitute coleslaw for the fries.

Classic Cheeseburger – A hefty all-beef patty seasoned and seared to perfection. Served with cheddar cheese, pickle planks, crisp lettuce and tomato, or go all out, and build your own. With a side of seasoned fries. I ask the waitperson to substitute green beans for the fries.

Burger Add-Ons

Cheddar Cheese.

Pepper Jack Cheese.

Sides:

Side salad.

Fresh coleslaw.

Green beans.

Lunch Combo:

A perfect lunch-sized portion of two favorite smoked meats, plus one side of your choice and a drink. Monday-Friday 11AM-4PM.

Smoked Chicken Breast – Boneless chicken breast marinated in our special seasoning mix, then smoked and sliced to order. Take a moment to savor the aroma before you dig in. Served with two sides of your choice.

Chopped Beef Brisket – Beef doesn't get any better than our smoked, hand-chopped brisket, slow-smoked for 12 hours. Served with any two sides.

Sliced Beef Brisket – Sliced is nice, too. Tender, smoked and seasoned with our BBQ spice . . . but not sliced until you order, so it's moist and full of flavor. Served with two sides of your choice.

BBQ Combos!

Pit Master's Choice – Brand new and really big. Our Pit

master's choice is plenty to eat with our chicken, chopped brisket, pulled pork and a rib, all smoked to perfection. Served with two sides of your choice. I ask the waitperson to ask the chef to substitute extra chicken and brisket for the pulled pork and the rib.

Create Your Own: - Can't decide? Choose from any of our tender smoked meats to create your own tasty platter. Served with two sides of your choice.

Three-meat combo.

Two meat combo.

Pit choices:

Chopped brisket.

Chicken breast.

Smoked turkey.

Sliced brisket.

Romano's Macaroni Grill

Chain Restaurant

Italian Tapas:

Spicy Ricotta Meatballs

Antipasti:

Pomodorina Soup – Plum tomatoes, mozzarella, crouton, basil pesto. I ask the waitperson to ask the chef to eliminate the croutons.

Blackboard Soup

Pantry:

Salad Sampler – Market chop, Caesar, Bibb & Blue. I ask the waitperson to ask the chef to substitute extra bib or bleu for the Caesar salad.

Caprese – Vine-ripened tomatoes, fresh mozzarella and basil.

Parmesan-Crusted Chicken – Fresh greens, prosciutto, parmesan ranch, balsamic glaze. I ask the waitperson to ask the chef to substitute extra fresh greens for the prosciutto.

Market Chop – Roasted turkey, pepperoni, provolone, artichoke, balsamic vinaigrette, and pumpkin seeds.

Bib & Blue – Bibb leaves, blue cheese, pancetta, walnuts, pickled red onions, buttermilk dressing. I ask the waitperson to ask the chef to substitute extra bib leaves for the pancetta.

Pollo:

Add fresh greens or bib and blue for an additional charge. Chicken is served with the skin on it. I cut the skin off.

Chicken Milanese – Argula parmesan salad, roasted potatoes, and lemon butter. I ask the waitperson to ask the chef to substitute green beans for the roasted potatoes.

Chicken Scaloppini – Artichokes, mushrooms, prosciutto, lemon butter, capellini. I ask the waitperson to ask the chef to leave the breading off the chicken, to substitute extra mushrooms for the prosciutto, and to substitute green beans for the capellini.

Pollo Caprese – Grilled chicken breast, capellini pomodoro, arugula salad. I ask the waitperson to ask the chef to substitute broccoli for the capellini pomodoro.

Grilled Chicken Spiedini –Roasted vegetables, lemon oil. I ask the waitperson to ask the chef to prepare this dish without the breading.

Chicken Under a Brick – Sage-roasted half chicken, asparagus, roasted potatoes, diavola sauce. I ask the waitperson to ask the chef to substitute extra asparagus for the roasted potatoes.

Chicken Marsala – Cremini mushrooms, marsala, sage, and capellini. I ask the waitperson to ask the chef to substitute green beans for the capellini.

Carne:

Add fresh greens or bib & blue for an additional charge.

Chianti BBQ Steak – Sirloin cap steak, prosciutto mac-n-cheese, grilled vegetables, garlic dip, and crostini. I ask the waitperson to ask the chef to substitute broccoli for the prosciutto mac-n-cheese and the crostini.

Parmesan-Crusted Veal Chop – Bone-in-scaloppini, prosciutto, mushroom & pea fettuccine, truffle demi-glace. I ask the waitperson to ask the waiter to substitute broccoli for the scaloppini and to substitute green beans for the fettuccine.

The Russian Tea Room

New York, NY

Because the same foods appear under a number of headings, in this section they are only listed once. They are listed as they first appeared on the menu.

Appetizers:

Traditional Tea Room Red Borscht – Pickled red beets, seasonable vegetables and dill in a short rib broth served with a braised beef pirozhok. I eat this appetizer on a reward night.

Onion Soup – Caramelized onion soup with gruyere and parmesan cheese and a crouton. I ask the waitperson to ask the chef to leave off the crouton.

Pelmeni Choice of braised beef pelmeni in a capon truffle consume with seasonal vegetables and mushrooms or Siberian style with cream, peas, and dill. I eat this appetizer on a reward night.

Salad Oliveier – Poached chicken, peas, potatoes, eggs, and roasted red peppers with a sour cream dill dressing. I eat this salad on a reward night.

Tea Room Market Salad – Shaved Jerusalem artichokes, grana padano cheese, pears and a tarragon vinaigrette dressing.

Grilled Eggplant Salad – Grilled eggplant and tomatoes marinated with extra virgin olive oil, oregano, vinegar and served with feta cheese and fresh mint. I ask the waitperson to ask the chef to leave off the mint.

Entrées:

Vegetable Tarelka – Mixed grilled vegetables with extra virgin olive oil and balsamic vinegar reduction.

Boeuf A La Stroganoff – Red wine braised beef short ribs with house-made buckwheat noodles tossed in a corn and black truffle cream sauce. I eat this entrée on a reward night.

Chicken Kiev – Herb butter stuffed in a breaded chicken breast with almond rice plov and mixed fruit chutney. I eat this dish on a reward night.

Hanger Steak – Chimichurri marinated hanger steak grilled, sliced, and served with a sweet potato and scallion hash. I ask the waitperson to ask the chef to substitute a vegetable for the sweet potato and scallion hash.

Kobe Burger – Grilled Kobe beef burger with grilled Vidalia onions and Maytag bleu cheese on a toasted garlic sourdough bread and served with sweet potato fries. I use the sourdough bread to drain off the juices and grease then discard it. I ask the waitperson to ask the chef to substitute a vegetable for the fries. I also request that bleu cheese be substituted for the Maytag bleu cheese.

Kobe Tasting Peringord – Kobe beef and American Grass-fed tasting with truffle mashed potatoes, asparagus with hollandaise and sauce au poivre. I ask the waitperson to ask the chef to substitute extra asparagus for the mashed potatoes.

Rack of Lamb – Pan seared rack of lamb, rutabaga and potato mash, sauteed Brussels sprouts in a cherry port reduction. I ask the waitperson to ask the chef to substitute vegetables for the rutabaga and potato mash.

Aged New York Strip – Dry aged New York strip steak with roasted garlic and fingerling potatoes. I ask the waitperson to ask the chef to substitute a vegetable for the potatoes.

Chicken A La Czar – Sauteed free-range chicken breast with mixed roasted peppers and mushrooms in a light cream sauce over spatzle. I eat this entrée on as reward night.

Shashlik Tasting – A tasting of the chef's special "shashlik" marinated beef, kefir curry marinated chicken, and chili-rubbed shrimp skewers served with fried panisse, courscous salad and spicy adjika. I ask the waitperson to ask the chef to substitute extra chicken for the shrimp. I eat this entrée on a reward night.

Desserts:

Chocolate Pyramid – bittersweet chocolate mousse with raspberry filing.

Famous Tea Room Blintzes – Cherry and cheese blintzes with vanilla ice cream.

Chocolate Mi-Cuit – Chocolate cake with a molten center, cherry ice cream, and a Grand Mariner cherry sauce.

Crème Brulee – Lavender honey vanilla crème brulee with mixed berries.

Express Lunch (starters, main course) and Dinner (appetizers, entrées) contain the same courses as listed above. The only editions to the dinner menu are:

Starters:

Goat Cheese and Wild Mushroom Blinchik – Crepe filled with mixed mushroooms and melted onions topped with lingonberries.

Brunch:

Russian Yogurt – Fresh berries and spiced almonds. I eat this dish on a reward day.

Fruit Plate – Chef's selection of seasonal fruit.

Eggs:

Golden Egg White Omelette – Spinach with sauteed mushrooms and gruyere cheese.

RTR Cobb Salad – Balsamic Marinated chicken breast grilled atop traditional Cobb salad. I ask the waitperson to ask the chef to substitute extra vegetables for the bacon and avocado.

Steak And Eggs – 10-ounce sirloin steak topped with sunny side eggs and foie gras potato hash. I ask the waitperson to ask the chef to substitute a vegetable for the foie gras potato hash.

Ruth's Chris Steak House

Chain Restaurant

Salads:

<u>Steak House Salad</u> – Iceberg, baby arugula, and baby lettuces with grape tomatoes, garlic croutons, and red onions. I ask the waitperson to ask the chef to leave off the croutons.

<u>Ruth's Chop Salad</u> – A Ruth Chris original, julienne iceberg lettuce, spinach and radicchio tossed with red onions and mushrooms, green olives, bacon eggs, hearts of palm, croutons, bleu cheese crumbles and lemon basil dressing. Topped with crispy fried onions. I ask the waitperson to ask the chef to substitute extra spinach and mushrooms for the bacon and crispy fried onions.

<u>Caesar Salad</u> – Fresh crisp romaine hearts tossed with Romano cheese and a creamy Caesar dressing. Topped with shaved parmesan cheese and fresh black pepper. I ask the waitperson to ask the chef to substitute bleu cheese dressing for the Caesar dressing.

<u>Lettuce Wedge</u> – A crisp wedge of iceberg lettuce on field greens topped with bacon, bleu cheese and your choice of dressing. I ask the waitperson to ask the chef to leave off the bacon.

<u>Vine Ripe Tomato & Mozzarella Salad</u> – A sliced beefsteak tomato with basil and fresh mozzarella cheese, served with balsamic vinaigrette.

Entrées:

<u>Filet</u> – the most tender cut of corn-fed Midwestern beef.

<u>Petite Filet</u> – A smaller, but equally tender filet.

<u>New York Strip</u> – This USA cut has a full-bodied texture that is slightly firmer than a Ribeye.

T-Bone- A full-flavored classic cut of USDA Prime cut.

Cowboy Ribeye – A huge bone-in version of this USDA Prime cut.

Porterhouse for Two – This USDA Prime cut combines the rich flavor of a strip with the tenderness of a filet.

Lamb Chops – Three chops cut extra thick, marinated overnight and served with fresh mint. They are naturally tender and flavorful.

Stuffed Chicken Breast – Oven-roasted double chicken breast stuffed with garlic herb cheese and served with lemon butter.

Dessert:

Crème Brulee – The classic Creole egg custard, topped with fresh berries and mint.

Bread Pudding with Whiskey Sauce – Our definitive version of a traditional New Orleans favorite.

Saltgrass Steak House

Chain Restaurant

Appetizers:

Artichoke & Spinach Dip – Served with tostada chips and salsa. I do not eat the chips.

Soups & Salads:

Our homemade salad dressings are honey-mustard, chunky bleu cheese, ranch & balsamic vinaigrette. Served with our Shiner Bock Beer Bread. I ask the waitperson to ask the chef to leave the bacon and croutons off all salads.

Great Soups Made Daily – Chicken tortilla or steak soup. I ask the waitperson to ask the chef to leave the tortilla strips off the chicken tortilla soup.

Soup & Salad – A bowl of your choice of soup with our Caesar or House Salad with crisp greens covered with bacon, eggs, croutons, grated cheese, & tomatoes. I ask the waitperson to substitute bleu cheese dressing for the Caesar dressing.

Grilled Chicken Salad - Grilled chicken breast strips on our Caesar or a bed of crisp greens with tortilla strips, bacon, eggs, croutons, & tomatoes. I ask the waitperson to ask the chef to leave off the tortilla strips and to substitute bleu cheese for the Caesar dressing.

Tenderloin Cobb Salad – Beef tenderloin tips grilled & sliced over crisp greens with chopped eggs, bacon, bleu cheese crumbles diced tomatoes, black olives & sliced avocados. I ask the waitperson to ask the chef to substitute extra diced tomatoes for the avocados.

Steak Salad – Certified Angus beef top sirloin grilled & thinly sliced over crisp greens with red potatoes, green beans, black olives, onions, tomato, bleu cheese crumbles, tossed with our balsamic vinaigrette. I ask the waitperson to ask the chef to substitute extra tomatoes for the red potatoes.

Sandwiches & Burgers:

Burgers and sandwiches are served with French fries. Add a dinner salad, Caesar salad, spinach salad, or a cup of soup for an extra charge. On all burgers and sandwiches I ask the waitperson to ask the chef to substitute a dinner salad for the French fries.

Cheeseburger – Half pound of grilled certified Angus beef fresh ground chuck with cheddar cheese, served with lettuce, tomato, onion & pickles on our homemade bun.

Chicken Sandwich – Grilled chicken breast, melted Jack cheese, crisp bacon, lettuce, tomato, onion, & pickles on our homemade bun with honey-mustard. I ask the waitperson to ask the chef to substitute extra tomato for the bacon.

Texas Cheesesteak Sandwich – Shaved certified Angus beef strip steak, grilled onions & poblano pepper topped with melted Jack cheese on a French roll with chipotle sauce.

Steaks:

We proudly serve certified Angus beef, known for its superior quality, tenderness & flavor. Our steaks are seasoned with our Saltgrass-7-Steak Spice & topped with garlic butter. Served with a dinner salad, Caesar salad, or a cup of soup & Shiner Bock Beer Bread plus your choice of a side. Substitute a spinach salad or asparagus for an extra charge. I do not eat the bread.

Wagon Boss Top Sirloin – Certified Angus beef center cut top sirloin, lean & full of flavor.

Cattleman's Prime Rib – Certified Angus prime rib, herb crusted & slow roasted for tenderness. Served with au jus.

Pat's Ribeye – Certified Angus beef Ribeye is our most flavorful steak.

New York Strip – Certified Angus beef center cut steak. The choice of the "Urban Cowboy".

Silver Star Porterhouse – Certified Angus beef Porterhouse is two steaks in one. Featuring ample portions of both filet & strip enhanced with "bone-in" flavor.

Cowboy Ribeye – Certified Angus beef bone-in Ribeye is our most flavorful steak. You better be hungry!

Maudeen's Center Cut Filet – Our most tender steak! Signature center cut filet mignon, perfectly lean, served thick and juicy.

Great Steak Additions:

Pepper crusted with cognac pepper or creamy peppercorn sauce.

Bleu cheese butter.

Sautéed mushrooms & grilled onion combo.

Sautéed mushrooms.

Saltgrass Favorites:

Chopped Sirloin Steak – Certified Angus beef ground steak topped with grilled onions, cheddar cheese & diced tomatoes or grilled onions, sautéed mushrooms & cognac pepper sauce.

Saltgrass K-Bob – beef tenderloin medallions grilled with fresh vegetables & paired with two bacon wrapped shrimp & chicken brochette. I ask the waitperson to ask the chef to substitute extra chicken brochette for the bacon wrapped shrimp.

Grilled Chicken Breast – Marinated grilled boneless chicken breast.

Hickory Chicken – Marinated grilled boneless chicken breast brushed with our BBQ sauce & topped with sautéed mushrooms & melted Jack cheese.

Brazos Chicken – Grilled chicken topped with Texas goat cheese, sundried tomatoes & ancho chipotle sauce. Served with garlic mashed potatoes. I ask the waitperson to ask the chef to substitute a small dinner salad for the mashed potatoes.

El Paso Chicken – Marinated grilled boneless chicken breast topped with roasted tomato salsa, melted Jack cheese, poblano pepper & pico de gallo

Sides:

Seasonal Veggies.

Asparagus.

Schlafly Bottleworks

Maplewood, MO

Please note that our menu changes seasonally and some items may not be available.

Appetizers:

<u>Meat & Cheese Platter</u> – Artisanal meats and cheeses, seasonal jam, smoked garlic and toast points. I do not eat the jam or toast points.

<u>Goat Cheese Dip</u> – Toasted pita, curry crackers. I do not eat the pita or crackers.

Salads:

<u>Field Green</u> – Spring mix, goat cheese, toasted almond, croutons, Vanilla vinaigrette. I ask the waitperson to ask the chef to substitute extra greens for the croutons.

<u>Greens & Grains</u> – Grain blend, spring mix, baked chicken, Sun-Dried Tomato Ranch. I ask the waitperson to ask the chef to substitute extra spring mix for the grain blend.

<u>Italian</u> – Spring mix, house blend, kalamata olives, red onion, White Balsamic Vinegar.

<u>Soup & Salad</u> – Half portion of any salad and a cup of soup.

<u>Housemade Dressings</u> – Vanilla Vinaigrette, Italian, and Sun-Dried Tomato Ranch.

Add grilled chicken or roasted mushrooms to any salad for an additional charge.

Soups:

<u>Soup of the Day</u> – Our chef's fresh-made daily soup.

<u>Beer Cheese</u> – Creamy white cheddar and dry Hopped PA.

<u>Vegetable Barley Stew</u> – Black barley and vegetable soup. My husband eats this stew.

Pizzas:

Bottleworks pizzas are about 10" and start with our hand-tossed Pilsner dough (gluten-free also available). Half-sized pizzas are also available. My husband and I share one pizza.

Herbivore – Green peppers, red onions, kalamata olives, spinach, mushrooms red sauce and house blend cheese.

Formaggiovore – All of our cheese toppings, your choice of sauce.

Veggie Toppings – Green peppers, roasted garlic, mushrooms, kalamata olives, onions, sun-dried tomatoes, and spinach.

Sauces – Rich tomato, smoked gouda cream, garlic oil, and BBQ.

Cheeses – House blend (mozzarella, smoked gouda, provolone, Jack and cheddar) feta, goat, and mozzarella.

Sandwiches:

Smoked Turkey – Smoked turkey, bacon, honey mustard, provolone and lettuce on griddled bistro with a side of slaw. I ask the waitperson to ask the chef to substitute extra provolone for the bacon.

Bison Burger – 8 oz. bison on a toasted brioche bun with a side of slaw.

Grilled Chicken – Grilled beer-brined chicken breast, Swiss, side of honey mustard on a toasted brioche bun with a side of slaw.

Turkey Burger – Turkey burger on a toasted wheat bun with spinach, brie and tomato-mint jam with a side of slaw. I ask the waitperson to ask the chef to substitute honey mustard for the tomato-mint jam.

Grilled Portobello – Grilled Portobello, provolone, spinach, roasted garlic-green olive mayo on a wheat bun with a side of grain blend. I ask the waitperson to ask the chef to substitute slaw for the grain blend.

Add Swiss, provolone, cheddar, blue, Gouda, pepper Jack or Jack cheese to any cold or hot sandwich for an additional charge.

Entrées:

Grass Fed Ribeye – 12 oz. grilled Ribeye finished with roasted garlic chive butter. Served with grilled asparagus and potato gratin. I ask the waitperson to ask the chef to substitute sautéed vegetables for the potato gratin.

Sides:

Grilled Asparagus.

Slaw.

Smoked Gouda Gratin.

Sautéed Vegetables.

Sautéed Spinach.

Dessert:

Sticky Toffee Pudding – Pudding in the Scottish sense – a very moist, dense cake; served with warm caramel sauce and freshly whipped cream.

Imperial Stout Pecan Pie – Northern Missouri pecans and Schlafly Imperial Stout.

Tahoe Joe's

Chain Restaurant

All salads and green beans contain bacon.

Appetizers:

Spinach & Artichoke Dip – A rich and creamy four-cheese blend with fresh spinach and artichoke hearts served with wood roasted salsa and crisp tortilla chips. I do not eat the tortilla chips.

Sierra Mountain Specialties:

Add a mixed green salad, baby greens salad or a bowl of homemade soup for an additional charge.

Joe's-Style Roasted Chicken – A half chicken, seasoned with Joe's proprietary spices, slow roasted and finished on our almond wood grill. Paired with Mountain Mashers and Blue Lake Green Beans. I ask the waitperson to ask the chef to substitute steamed vegetables for the Mountain Mashers and Blue Lake Green Beans.

Wood Grilled Chicken – Whiskey Peppercorn or BBQ Glazed. Served with Mountain Mashers and Blue Lake Green Beans. I ask the waitperson to ask the chef to substitute a big salad without the bacon for the Mountain Mashers and the Blue Lake Green Beans.

Whiskey Peppercorn Sirloin – Slow-roasted Joe's Steak® sliced and topped with a whiskey cream sauce. Served with Mountain Mashers and Blue Lake Green Beans. I ask the waitperson to ask the chef to substitute steamed vegetables for the Mountain Mashers and the Blue Lake Green Beans.

Joe's Bowls:

Joe's Steak® Salad – Thinly-sliced Joe's Steak® tops this hearty salad of baby field greens tossed with a light Champagne Vinaigrette, sweet walnuts, tomatoes and

Gorgonzola cheese. I ask the waitperson to ask the chef to leave off the bacon.

Citrus Chicken Salad – Baby field greens, wood grilled chicken, Gorgonzola cheese, fresh avocado and cucumber tossed in our Citrus Vinaigrette topped with sweet walnuts. Mandarin oranges and crisp wonton strips. I ask the waitperson to ask the chef to substitute extra baby field greens for the avocado, cucumber, bacon, and crisp wonton strips.

Wood Grilled Chicken Salad – Hand-pulled chicken atop baby field greens tossed with a light Champagne Vinaigrette, raisins, sweet walnuts, tomatoes, and Gorgonzola cheese. I ask the waitperson to ask the chef to leave the bacon off.

Joe's Steak® Sandwich – Hand-carved Joe's Steak®, mushrooms, onions, tomatoes, bacon, cheese, a green chili, and Thousand Island dressing between grilled Parmesan bread. I ask the waitperson to ask the chef to leave off the bacon and to substitute bleu cheese dressing for the Thousand Island dressing. I eat this on a reward night.

Black Jack Burger – Half pound of wood grilled Angus beef topped with crisp bacon and your choice of cheese. I ask the waitperson to ask the chef to substitute extra cheese for the bacon.

Wood Grilled Steaks:

Our steaks are grilled over real almond wood fire. We use only mid-western, corn-fed beef aged a minimum of 28 days.

Choice of One – Baby greens salad, mixed greens salad, Caesar salad (I substitute bleu cheese dressing for the Caesar dressing), or homemade soup.

Choice of One – Because I do not eat the rice of potatoes I ask the waitperson to ask the chef to give me an extra serving of one of the above choices.

Joe's Ribeye – 14 oz. Our most popular cut. Try the 20 oz. Nebraska.

Ponderosa Sirloin – A thick 12 oz. cut.

Joe's Steak® - Our slow roasted sirloin rolled in cracked black pepper and wood grilled.

Twin Petite Filets – Two 5 oz. bacon-wrapped filets topped with your choice of garlic butter or Gorgonzola cheese. I ask the waitperson to ask the chef to remove the bacon before cooking my steak.

New York Strip – 14 oz. choice cut.

Sierra Steak – 9 oz. marinated sirloin.

Tahoe T-Bone – A 22 oz. choice cut featuring the New York and Filet.

Cabin Combos:

Our signature 6 oz. Joe's Steak® paired with one of your favorites. I order the wood grilled BBQ chicken.

Joe's Steak Mushrooms – Found only at Tahoe Joe's. Simmered in white wine, butter and au jus with just a hint of garlic. Add to any entrée for an additional charge.

Prime Rib:

Rubbed with fresh Rosemary and Joe's special blend of spices then show-roasted for maximum flavor and tenderness. Includes your choice of soup or salad and a scratch made side.

Lunch:

See Joe's Bowls above.

Unlimited Soup and Salad – Scratch-made soup, signature salads and fresh-baked sourdough rolls.

Campfire Burgers & Sandwiches:

All burgers & sandwiches are served with hand-cut Cabin

Fries. I ask the waitperson to ask the chef to substitute a small dinner salad or steamed vegetables for the fries.

Joe's Steak® Sandwich – Hand-cut Joe's Steak®, mushrooms, onions, tomatoes, crisp bacon, Jack cheese, Thousand Island dressing and a green chili between grilled Parmesan bread. I ask the waitperson to ask the chef to substitute extra onions for the bacon and bleu cheese dressing for the Thousand Island dressing. I eat this sandwich on a reward night.

Mushroom Burger – Tender mushrooms and Jack cheese make this half pound wood grilled burger a must.

California Chicken Sandwich – A wood grilled chicken breast topped with Jack cheese and crisp bacon along with fresh sliced avocado. Honey mustard dressing, lettuce and tomato. I ask the waitperson to ask the chef to substitute extra lettuce and tomato for the bacon and avocado.

Crystal Bay Chicken Sandwich - Wood grilled chicken, onions, mushrooms, fresh avocado and crisp bacon along with Jack cheese and green chili between grilled Parmesan bread. I ask the waitperson to ask the chef to substitute extra onions and mushrooms for the avocado and bacon. I eat this sandwich on a reward night.

Peppercorn Bleu Burger – Cracked black pepper and melted bleu cheese make this half pound Angus burger a winner.

Bacon Cheddar Burger – Half pound wood grilled Angus burger topped with cheddar cheese and crisp bacon. This burger is also served without bacon. I order it without the bacon.

Knife & Fork Mountain Dip – Thinly sliced and slow roasted steak topped with onions, mushrooms, and peppers and melted Jack cheese.

Sierra Mountain Specialties:

See list above.

Desserts:

<u>Ski Jump Chocolate Cake</u> – A rich double chocolate cake topped with fresh whipped cream and homemade chocolate sauce.

Texas Roadhouse

Chain Restaurant

Just for Starters:

Texas Red Chili – Made-from-scratch recipe, topped with cheddar cheese and red onions.

Salads:

All salads served with your choice of made-from-scratch dressing: Ranch, Honey Mustard, Italian, and Bleu cheese.

Grilled Chicken Salad – Crisp cold greens, strips of marinated chicken, Jack cheese, egg, tomato, bacon, red onions, and croutons. I ask the waitperson to ask the chef to substitute extra tomato for the bacon and croutons.

Chicken Caesar Salad – Tender strips of grilled chicken tossed with hearts of romaine, fresh parmesan cheese, made-from-scratch croutons, and our zesty Caesar dressing. I ask the waitperson to ask the chef to substitute extra hearts of romaine for the croutons and bleu cheese dressing for the Caesar dressing.

Chicken Critter® Salad – Hot crispy strips of chicken piled high on a bed of cold greens with Jack and cheddar cheeses, egg, tomato, and bacon. I ask the waitperson to ask the chef to substitute grilled chicken for the crispy chicken strips and to substitute extra greens for the bacon.

Steakhouse Filet Salad – Salad greens drizzled with Italian dressing, topped with tender filet strips, bleu cheese crumbles, bacon bits, red onions, tomatoes, and croutons, and served with a side of creamy bleu cheese. I ask the waitperson to ask the chef to substitute extra tomatoes for the bacon bits and to substitute extra red onion for the croutons.

House Salad – Fresh greens, cheddar cheese, tomato, eggs,

and made-from-scratch croutons. I ask the waitperson to ask the chef to substitute extra tomato for the croutons.

Hand-Cut Steaks:

Each plate served with your choice of two sides. For an extra charge you can smother your steak with sautéed mushrooms or Jack cheese.

USDA Choice Sirloin – 6 oz., 8oz., 11 oz. Hearty Cut, or 16 oz. Cowboy Cut.

New York Strip of Ft. Worth Ribeye – 10 oz., 12 oz. or 16 oz.

Bone-In Ribeye – Our largest and most flavorful steak, hand – cut to perfection. 20 oz.

Texas T-Bone – 18 oz.

Dallas Filet – 6oz. or 8oz.

Filet Medallions – Three tender filets (9 oz. total) topped with choice of Peppercorn or Portobello mushroom sauce and served over seasoned rice. I ask the waitperson to ask the chef to substitute green beans for the rice.

Road Kill – 10 oz. chopped steak smothered with sautéed onions, sautéed mushrooms, and Jack cheese.

Sirloin Kabob – Marinated sirloin with onion, mushroom, tomato, red and green peppers, served on a bed of seasoned rice (choice of one side). I order green beans and ask the waitperson to ask the chef to substitute a house salad for the rice.

Prime Rib – Please ask us about availability. Horseradish upon request. 10 oz., 12 oz., or 16 oz.

Chicken Specialties:

Each plate is served with your choice of two sides.

Grilled BBQ Chicken – Marinated ½ lb. breast basted in our BBQ sauce.

Oven Roasted Chicken – Half chicken trimmed, uniquely

seasoned and slow roasted to the perfect tenderness.

Smothered Chicken – Grilled, marinated chicken breast with sautéed onions, sautéed mushrooms and made-from-scratch gravy or Jack cheese. I order the Jack cheese.

Portobello Mushroom Chicken – Marinated chicken breast grilled and topped with Portobello Mushroom sauce, Jack cheese and fresh parmesan.

Country Dinners:

Each plate is served with your choice of two sides.

Sirloin Beef Tips – Sirloin pieces, sautéed mushrooms, onions, brown gravy and sour cream served over seasoned rice or mashed potatoes (choice of one side). I order the house salad and ask the waitperson to ask the chef to substitute green beans for the rice or potatoes.

Country Veg Plate – Choose a total of 4 side items (only one salad). I order the house salad, fresh vegetables, green beans, and cup of chili.

Legendary Sides/Extras:

Cup of Chili.

House Salad.

Caesar Salad – I ask the waitperson to ask the chef to substitute bleu cheese dressing for the Caesar dressing.

Fresh Vegetables.

Green Beans.

Sautéed Onions.

Sautéed Mushrooms.

Burgers & Sandwiches:

Served on a toasted Texas-sized bun with steak fries and a pickle spear. I ask the waitperson to ask the chef to substitute a house salad or green beans for the steak fries.

<u>Burgers</u> – 1/2 lb. fresh ground chuck with lettuce, tomato, and onion.

<u>All-American Cheeseburger</u> – Our classic with American cheese. I ask the waitperson to ask the chef to substitute cheddar or Swiss cheese for the American cheese.

<u>Smokehouse Burger</u> – Sautéed mushrooms, onions and BBQ sauce with American and Jack cheeses. I ask the waitperson to substitute extra Jack cheese for the American cheese.

<u>BBQ Chicken</u> – Marinated and grilled, then basted with BBQ sauce and served with lettuce, tomato, and onion.

<u>Mushroom Jack Chicken</u> – Fresh chicken breast with sautéed mushrooms, melted Jack cheese, and served with lettuce, tomato, and onion.

Desserts:

Granny's Apple Classic.

Strawberry Cheesecake.

Big Ol' Brownie.

Early Dine:

Mon-Thurs. Until 6 PM – Come in early and chose from 10 dinners at a great price:

6 oz. Sirloin Steak.

10 oz. Road Kill Chopped Steak.

Grilled BBQ Chicken.

Grilled Chicken Salad.

Chicken Caesar Salad – I ask the waitperson to ask the chef to substitute bleu cheese dressing for the Caesar dressing.

Weck's

Albuquerque, Santa Fe, Rio Rancho, and Los Lunas, NM

"Full Belly" Omelettes:

Four eggs served with fresh hash browns, toast or tortilla. On all Omelettes I ask the waitperson to ask the chef to substitute extra vegetables for the hash browns and the toast/tortillas.

Farmers Market – Sautéed mushrooms, onions, bell peppers, sprouts, diced tomatoes, and guacamole, sour cream, and cheddar and Jack cheeses, with your choice of red and/or green chili. I ask the waitperson to ask the chef to substitute extra cheddar for the guacamole.

The Abney – Diced bacon, fresh bell peppers, diced tomatoes, and guacamole, cheddar and Jack cheeses, with your choice of red and/or green chili. I ask the waitperson to ask the chef to substitute extra bell peppers and tomatoes for the bacon and the guacamole.

Healthier Alternative – Fresh onions, mushrooms, bell peppers, sprouts, and diced tomatoes folded into cholesterol-free egg substitute, eggs or egg whites topped with fresh diced green chili and served with sliced tomatoes and dry toast. (Veggies are served uncooked.) I order the eggs.

South of Denver Omelette – Diced ham, sautéed bell peppers and onions with cheddar and Jack cheeses and your choice of red and/or green chili. I ask the waitperson to ask the chef to substitute diced tomatoes for the diced ham.

Build Your Own Omelette – Start with a fluffy four egg Omelette and a blend of cheddar and Jack cheeses with your choice of red and/or green chili. Add your favorite ingredients (additional charge). Bell pepper, sautéed mushrooms, chopped green chili, sautéed onions, diced tomatoes, sprouts or sour cream.

Big Sandwiches:

All sandwiches are served with your choice of any two: fresh fruit, cottage cheese, or substitute a small salad or bowl of soup for both sides.

<u>T.G.G.</u> – Turkey, fresh green chili, guacamole, bacon, mozzarella cheese, lettuce and tomato on griddled whole wheat. I ask the waitperson to ask the chef to substitute extra mozzarella cheese and tomatoes for the bacon and guacamole.

<u>Spicy Reuben</u> – Corned beef, turkey, kraut, Swiss cheese and fresh green chili on griddled rye.

<u>Different Philly</u> – Your choice of roast beef or turkey, sautéed mushrooms, onions, bell pepper and mozzarella cheese on griddled sourdough.

<u>Chicken Club</u> – Charbroiled chicken breast with fresh green chili, bacon, cheddar cheese, lettuce and tomato on toasted multi-grain bread. I ask the waitperson to ask the chef to substitute extra lettuce and tomato for the bacon and to leave off the middle slice of bread.

<u>Funky Chicken</u> – Charbroiled chicken breast, sautéed mushrooms, onions, fresh green chili, bacon and Swiss cheese on griddled sourdough. I ask the waitperson to ask the chef to substitute extra Swiss cheese for the bacon.

Belly Bustin' Burgers:

All of our burgers are one half pound of the finest USDA choice lean ground beef, served on a toasted specialty bun with lettuce, tomato, onion and pickle chips. I ask the waitperson to ask the chef to substitute extra lettuce and tomatoes for the wedge fries or potato chips.

<u>Hamburger.</u>

<u>Cheeseburger.</u>

Green Chile Cheeseburger.

Frisco Burger – One half pound patty, sautéed onions, topped with melted cheddar cheese, lettuce, tomato and homemade Frisco sauce on two slices of grilled sourdough. I order it served open faced.

Build Your Own Burger – Start with a delicious half pound patty and add cheese (Cheddar or Swiss), fresh green chili, or sautéed mushrooms. (An additional charge per item.)

Open Faced Green Chili Burger – A mouth-watering burger served open faced and smothered with green chili sauce and cheddar and Jack cheeses.

Big Salads & Soups:

Salads are served with a fresh multi-grain roll and choice of dressing.

Santa Fe – Charbroiled diced chicken breast, fresh green chili, cheddar and Jack cheeses, diced tomatoes, black olives, cucumbers, carrots, bell peppers, croutons and sunflower seeds atop a bed of our Romaine lettuce. I ask the waitperson to ask the chef to substitute extra diced tomatoes and bell peppers for the cucumbers and croutons.

The Anderson – Diced fresh smoked turkey, guacamole, diced bacon, cheddar and Jack cheeses, tomatoes, cucumbers, carrots, bell peppers, croutons and sunflower seeds atop a bed of our Romaine lettuce. I ask the waitperson to ask the chef to substitute extra Romaine lettuce and tomatoes for the diced bacon, cucumbers, and croutons.

Chicken Salad – Large dollop of scratch made chicken salad, Parmesan cheese, tomatoes, cucumbers, carrots, almonds and sunflower seeds atop a bed of our Romaine lettuce. I ask the waitperson to ask the chef to substitute extra tomatoes for the cucumbers.

Fresh Garden Salad – Cheddar and Jack cheeses, tomatoes, cucumbers, carrots, bell peppers, croutons and sunflower seeds atop a bed of our Romaine lettuce. I ask the waitperson to ask the chef to substitute extra Romaine lettuce for the cucumbers and croutons.

Weck's Green Chile Chicken Stew – Scratch made stew made with tender chicken and fresh green chili. Served with a tortilla.

Soup of the Day – Changes daily. Ask your server about today's soup.

On the Lighter Side:

A special selection of healthier alternatives and vegetarian choices!

Fresh Turkey – Fresh smoked turkey, Swiss cheese, guacamole, sprouts, lettuce and tomato on a lightly grilled croissant. Served with a small salad. I ask the waitperson to ask the chef to substitute extra Swiss cheese for the guacamole.

Veggie Delight – Cream cheese, almonds, sunflower seeds, guacamole, cucumbers, bell peppers, carrots, lettuce, tomato and sprouts on toasted multi-grain bread. Served with a small salad. I ask the waitperson to ask the chef to substitute extra bell peppers and tomatoes for the guacamole and cucumbers.

Chicken Salad – Scratch made chicken salad with cheddar cheese, lettuce and tomato on a lightly grilled croissant. Served with a small salad.

Scratch Made Soup and Small Salad – Served with a fresh multi-grain roll.

Sides:

Fresh Fruit (Seasonal).

Salsa.

Chile (red, green, or chopped green.)

Small Salad – Tomatoes, cucumbers, carrots, bell peppers, croutons and sunflower seeds atop a bed of our Romaine lettuce. I ask the waitperson to ask the chef to substitute extra Romaine lettuce and tomatoes for the cucumbers and croutons.

Ya Ya's

Euro Bistro
Chain Restaurant

Dinner:
Meat and Poultry:

Chicken Pizzetta – Marsala, caramelized onions, Ya Ya's cheese blend, mushrooms and thyme.

Tavern Pita – Choice of spiced free range chicken or grilled grass fed beef, with warm pita, Greek yogurt, and harissa.

Beef Carpaccio - Goat cheese, white truffle oil, baby arugula, oven-dried tomatoes, fried capers, and crisps.

Oak Fired Pizzas:

Four Cheeses – Provolone, house made mozzarella, fontina, parmesan, marinara, and basil pesto.

Chicken Piadini – Flatbread, roasted chicken, bell peppers, feta, hummus, and red chili oil.

Free Range Chicken & Mushrooms – Farmstead cheddar, bell peppers, tomatoes, and red onions.

Greens:

Bill's Chicken Salad – Hot mustard glazed crispy chicken tenders, mixed greens, avocado, egg, tomato, cheese, artichoke hearts, and balsamic vinaigrette. I ask the waitperson to ask the chef to substitute extra tomato for the avocado.

Market Salad – Mixed field greens, kalamata olives, cucumber, red onion and lemon vinaigrette. Add grilled chicken for an additional charge. I ask the waitperson to ask the chef to substitute extra red onion for the cucumbers.

Vegetable & Pita Salad – Fresh vegetables, greens, hearts of palm, kalamata olives, harissa, and eggplant yogurt on pita.

Add hickory grilled beef tenderloin or herb-roasted chicken for an additional charge.

Cobb Salad – Grilled chicken breast, romaine, bacon, tomatoes, gorgonzola, avocado, egg, radishes, red onion, and buttermilk dressing. I ask the waitperson to ask the chef to substitute extra tomatoes and red onion for the avocado and bacon.

Pastas:

Roasted Chicken Penne – Sweet peas, oven-dried tomatoes, parmesan, and roasted garlic cream. I eat this pasta on a reward night.

Lunch:
Same menu as the dinner menu.

Between Slices:

Grilled Beef Tenderloin – Roasted mushrooms, mozzarella, tomato jam, Dijon horseradish, fried onions on ciabatta. I ask the waitperson to ask the chef to substitute grilled onions for the fried onions.

Mr. Benne's Best Burger - Choice of cheese, traditional garnish, and fresh bun.

Pesto Chicken Salad – Fresh mozzarella, avocado, baby greens, red onion, tomato, and garlic aioli on wheat. I ask the waitperson to ask the chef to substitute extra red onion for the avocado.

Grilled Chicken Breast – Thick slab of bacon and cheddar cheese on a fresh bun, avocado aioli, lettuce, red onion, and tomato. I ask the waitperson to ask the chef to substitute extra tomato for the bacon.

Roasted Turkey – Bacon, lettuce, avocado, Monterey Jack, and blue cheese mayo, on peasant bread. I ask the waitperson to ask the chef to substitute tomato and red onion for the bacon and avocado.

Soup, Half Salad, or Half Sandwich – Choose two items.

Soups:

Tomato Vegetable.

Soup of the Day.

Zea Rotisserie Grill

Chain Restaurant

Appetizers:

Spinach Dip – Zea's twist on an American classic, topped with feta, corn chips for dipping. I do not eat the corn chips.

Soup Du Jour – a different selection daily.

Tomato Basil – Thursday.

Salads:

Spinach Salad – with pepper jelly vinaigrette, sun dried tomatoes, raisins, pecans, calamata olives bleu cheese, and sesame seeds. I ask the waitperson to ask the chef to substitute bleu cheese dressing for the pepper jelly vinaigrette.

House Salad – radicchio, carrots, tomato, Jack cheese and a choice of dressing. I ask the waitperson to ask the chef to substitute extra lettuce for the radicchio.

Almond Chicken Salad – Grilled chicken, crispy noodles, sesame seeds, herbs and peanut vinaigrette. I ask the waitperson to ask the chef to leave off the crispy noodles.

Rotisserie Meats and Poultry:

Served with your choice of two sides.

Zea Rotisserie Chicken - Seasoned and roasted half a chicken.

BBQ Chicken – Seasoned, roasted half a chicken, and glazed with zesty BBQ.

Sweet and Spicy Rotisserie Chicken – Seasoned, roasted half a chicken, with a sweet chile glaze.

Rotisserie Chicken & Meat of the Day Platter – half a chicken and a generous portion of today's meat.

Tuesday – Braised Provimi veal & Natural au jus.

Wednesday – Rotisserie beef with burgundy mushroom glace.

Thursday – Rotisserie Provimi leg of lamb & mustard mint demi-glace.

Saturday – Braised Provimi veal & Natural au jus.

Sunday - Rotisserie beef with burgundy mushroom glace.

From the Grill:

Served with your choice of two sides.

Ribeye Steak – Grilled to temperature and served with horseradish tiger sauce.

Zea Signature Prime Rib – Rotisseried, then grilled to temperature, and served with horseradish tiger sauce.

Wood Fire Chicken Breast – Seasoned and grilled over hardwood.

Tournedos of Filet – Twin 4 ounce beef tenderloin medallions seared and served with mushroom burgundy sauce.

Sides:

Single Serving.

Thai Snap Beans.

Vegetable Du Jour.

Sugar Snap Beans.

Substitute soup, house salad, or spinach salad for an additional charge.

Sandwiches:

Wood Fire Chicken Sandwich – Hickory grilled breast, Jack cheese, lettuce, tomato, and one side.

Zea Cheeseburger – A half pound of ground chuck, Jack, cheddar, or bleu cheese, lettuce, tomato and one side. Build your own! Mushrooms, grilled onions, BBQ sauce, or green chile available for an extra charge.

Zio's Italian Kitchen

Chain Restaurant

Appetizers:

Baked Formaggio – A blend of four cheeses and Italian herbs baked in our brick oven, topped with kalamata olive relish and served with grilled Italian bread.

Artichoke Spinach Dip – A blend of cheese, spinach, artichoke hearts, onions and bacon topped with Roma tomatoes and baked in our brick oven with Italian flat bread. I ask the waitperson to ask the chef to leave out the bacon.

Caprese Salad – Cool slices of vine-ripe tomatoes and dairy-fresh mozzarella cheese accented by flavorful fresh basil leaves and red onion. Drizzled with balsamic reduction and served with grilled Italian bread and Italian dressing.

Signature Soups and Salads:

All salads are served with your choice of dressing: homemade Italian, homemade ranch, bleu cheese, honey mustard, and homemade strawberry vinaigrette.

Soup of the Day – Please ask your server for details about today's selection.

Signature Soups – Tomato Florentine and Vegetable Minestrone.

Strawberry Field Salad – Romaine lettuce and spinach with slices of hot grilled chicken and sun-ripened strawberries. Topped with feta cheese and sugar glazed walnuts, then drizzled with homemade strawberry vinaigrette and served with grilled Italian flat bread. This dish contains tree nuts (walnuts).

Greek Chicken Salad – Baby spinach and Romaine tossed in our light balsamic vinaigrette dressing. Topped with hot grilled chicken, kalamata olives, feta cheese, fresh Roma tomatoes, and red onions.

House Italian Side Salad – Mixed greens, diced Roma tomatoes, artichoke hearts and parmesan. Garnished with pepperoncini and served with home style croutons and your choice of dressing. I ask the waitperson to ask the chef to substitute extra mixed greens for the croutons.

House Italian Dinner Salad – Mixed greens with diced Roma tomatoes, artichoke hearts and parmesan cheese. Garnished with pepperoncini and served with home style croutons and your choice of dressing. With grilled or Parmesan-crusted sliced chicken breast for an extra charge. I ask the waitperson to ask the chef to substitute extra mixed greens for the croutons.

Zio's Classic Pastas:

Add a house salad or a cup of our Signature soup for an additional charge.

Artichoke Spinach Pasta – Zio's artichoke spinach dip tossed with sliced chicken breast, bacon, onions, fresh Roma tomatoes and penne pasta. I ask the waitperson to ask the chef to substitute extra tomatoes for the bacon.

Pepperoni Chicken – Sliced chicken, pepperoni, grilled peppers and onions, fresh mushrooms, black olives and red pepper flakes sautéed, then tossed with penne pasta, marinara sauce and mozzarella cheese. I ask the waitperson to ask the chef to substitute extra grilled peppers and onions for the pepperoni.

Chicken Pomodoro – Sliced chicken breast, fresh garlic and basil, red pepper flakes sautéed in olive oil and white wine, then tossed with diced Roma tomatoes. Parmesan cheese and linguine.

Greek Pasta – Sliced chicken breast sautéed in a garlic, white wine and olive oil with kalamata olives, green onions, red pepper flakes and oregano. Tossed with penne, diced Roma tomatoes and feta cheese.

Lemon Chicken Primavera – Tender grilled chicken sautéed with broccoli, squash, carrots, mushrooms, red bell peppers, green olives, onion, zucchini, roasted garlic and red pepper flakes. Tossed in a light lemon olive oil and finished with penne pasta and a touch of Parmesan cheese.

Zio's House Specialties:

Add a house salad or a cup of our Signature soup for an extra charge.

Chicken Marsala – Grilled chicken breast topped with a Marsala wine pan sauce with red onions and mushrooms. Served with angel hair pasta or roasted rosemary potatoes. I ask the waitperson to ask the chef to substitute a vegetable for the pasta or potatoes.

Chicken Milanese – Pan-seared chicken breasts with fresh garlic, fresh mushrooms, diced Roma tomatoes and basil. Served on baby spinach with angel hair pasta in a lemon cream white wine.

Grilled Chicken Amalfi – A grilled chicken breast sautéed with mushrooms, green onions, red onions and sun-dried tomatoes in a delicate lemon cream sauce. Served with angel hair pasta. I ask the waitperson to ask the chef to substitute a vegetable for the pasta.

Vodka Chicken – A juicy, marinated and grilled chicken breast served atop angel hair pasta with spinach, prosciutto, black olives and creamy tomato vodka sauce. I ask the waitperson to ask the chef to substitute extra spinach for the prosciutto.

Chicken Piccata – Pan-seared chicken breasts sautéed with fresh baby spinach, mushrooms, artichoke hearts, prosciutto and capers. Finished in a lemon cream white wine sauce. Served over angel hair pasta. I ask the waitperson to ask the chef to substitute extra baby spinach for the prosciutto.

Grilled Sirloin – A juicy 9 oz. cut of sirloin grilled exactly to your liking. Served with roasted rosemary potatoes or seasonal vegetables. The plate is topped with a Parmesan mix. I order the seasonal vegetables.

Ribeye Tuscano – A 12 oz. seasoned Ribeye steak carefully grilled to your preference. Served with roasted rosemary potatoes or seasonal vegetables. The plate is topped with a Parmesan mix. I order the seasonal vegetables.

Sandwiches:

Sandwiches are served with your choice of House salad or a cup of our Signature soup.

Grilled Italian Chicken Sandwich – Grilled chicken breast, grilled onions, red and green bell peppers topped with smoked provolone cheese and garlic butter.

Chicken Parmigiana Sandwich - Our hand-breaded classic chicken Parmigiana topped with marinara, melted mozzarella and parmesan cheese. I ask the waitperson to ask the chef to substitute grilled chicken for the breaded chicken.

Pronto Lunches:

Monday-Friday 11am – 4pm. All lunch entrée orders include a House salad or a cup of our Signature soup.

Lunch entrées are smaller portions of previously listed entrées.

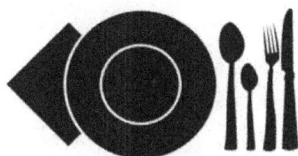

FAST FOOD RESTAURANTS

BREAKFAST

Grand Traverse Pie Company

Chain Restaurant

<u>Ham, Egg</u> and Cheese – Ham, egg, cheese and pesto mayo on your choice of bread. I ask the counterperson to ask the chef to substitute roasted red peppers for the ham.

<u>Breakfast Quiche</u> – Assorted varieties.

<u>Fresh Fruit Cup</u> – Select fresh cut fruits.

Paradise Bakery & Café/Panera/St. Louis Bread Company

Chain Restaurant

Paradise Bakery & Café's menu is not listed here because in the first edition of *FROM FAT TO FABULOUS: A DIET GUIDE FOR RESTAURANT LOVERS,* it is listed under St. Louis Bread Company/Panera Bread.

Building on the success of its Panera Cares program that allows diners to pay what they can for a meal, in select locations the company is now offering select meals at no set price. Diners can either pay the suggested price, pay more to cover the cost of someone else's meal, or pay what they can.

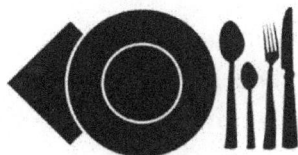

FAST FOOD RESTAURANTS

LUNCH/DINNER

Big A's

St. Charles, MO

Appetizers:

Spinach & Artichoke Dip – Fresh spinach and artichokes in a creamy sauce, with a platter of tortilla chips. I do not eat the tortilla chips.

Salads and Soups:

Dinner Salad – Lettuce, tomato, cucumber, mushrooms, red onion, Parmesan cheese, and croutons. I ask the waitperson to ask the chef to leave off the cucumber and croutons.

Specialty Chef Salad – Tomato, cucumber, red onion, cheese, egg, mushrooms, ham, turkey, and croutons. I ask the waitperson to ask the chef to leave off the cucumber, ham, and croutons.

Spinach Salad – Spinach, cucumber, tomato, sunflower seeds, almonds, bacon mozzarella cheese, with fajita chicken. I ask the waitperson to ask the chef to leave off the cucumber and the bacon.

Italian Salad – Red onion, tomato, black olives, cucumbers, and Parmesan cheese. I ask the waitperson to ask the chef to leave off the cucumbers.

Chicken Caesar Salad – Lettuce, Parmesan cheese and croutons tossed in a Caesar dressing, with fajita chicken. I ask the waitperson to ask the chef to leave off the croutons and to substitute blue cheese dressing for the Caesar dressing.

Chicken Salad – Grilled chicken marinated in Italian Dijon blend with onions, tomato, and cheese. Served in a shell. I ask the waitperson to ask the chef to substitute extra vegetables for the shell.

Buffalo Chicken Salad – grilled or breaded chicken marinated in hot sauce, with lettuce, onions, tomato, and cheese. Served in a shell. I order the chicken grilled and ask the waitperson to ask the chef to substitute extra vegetables for the shell.

<u>Salad Dressings</u> – Italian, French, bleu cheese, honey Dijon, and Balsamic Vinaigrette.

<u>Soups</u> – Beer cheese soup or soup of the day. Served in a cup or a bowl.

<u>Burgers:</u>

All burgers are made of extra lean USDA Angus ground chuck and grilled to perfection. Served on a sesame seed bun with pickle spear and your choice of one side. Cole slaw or steamed broccoli. For an extra charge you can substitute a dinner salad or a cup of soup. On all burgers I used the bun to drain off the extra juices and the grease, and I discard the bun.

<u>The Big A's 8oz Burger</u> – For an extra charge you can add

Cheddar or Swiss cheese.

<u>The Little A's 4 oz. Burger</u> – For an extra charge you can add Cheddar, Swiss, Mozzarella, or jalapeno cheese.

<u>Main Street Favorite</u> – Sauteed mushrooms and cheese.

<u>Bleu Cheese</u> – Covered in bleu cheese crumbles.

<u>Entrées:</u>

Fresh steaks, hand-cut and grilled to perfection and topped with homemade garlic steak butter, served with a dinner salad, and a choice of a side. Served after 5:00 p.m.

<u>12 oz Charbroiled Ribeye.</u>

<u>9 oz Center-Cut</u> – Bacon wrapped filet mignon. I ask the waitperson to ask the chef to prepare my steak without the bacon.

Boston Market

Chain Restaurant

Individual Meals:

Our home style individual meals are served with your choice of two regular gourmet sides and cornbread. I do not eat the cornbread.

Rotisserie Chicken Meals –

Chose from original, BBQ, or spicy sauces for a flavorful kick. I do not use any of the sauces.

Half Chicken.

Quarter White.

Three Piece Dark.

Home Style Plates

Turkey Breast.

Beef Brisket.

Meatloaf.

Sandwiches & Salads

Boston Market sandwiches are made fresh for you and are topped with lettuce and tomato. Our entrée salads are tossed to order and served with our delicious cornbread. I do not eat the cornbread. I order all sandwiches open faced. I use the bottom bun to drain off the juices and grease, and discard it.

Rotisserie Chicken Carver ® - With lettuce, tomatoes, Dijon mustard, vinaigrette, and cheese.

All-White Rotisserie Chicken Salad – With mayo, celery, lettuce, tomatoes, and vinaigrette.

Turkey Carver ® - With lettuce, tomatoes, dill parmesan mayo, vinaigrette, and cheese.

Meatloaf Carver ® - With lettuce, tomatoes, hickory ketchup, and cheese. I ask the waitperson to substitute Dijon mustard for the hickory ketchup.

Brisket Dip Carver ® - With mayo, cheese, and au jus.

Hand-Tossed Salads:

Mediterranean Salad – Rotisserie chicken, mixed greens, feta, tomatoes, cucumbers, onions, and sweet garlic vinaigrette. I ask the waitperson to leave off the cucumbers.

Southwest Santa Fe Salad – Rotisserie chicken, mixed greens, corn, poblano pepper and black bean relish, tomatoes, onions, tortilla strips, cheddar cheese, and chipotle cheddar dressing. I ask the waitperson to substitute extra mixed greens and tomatoes for corn, black bean relish, and tortilla strips.

Caesar Salad – Rotisserie chicken, romaine, an Italian blend of cheeses, and croutons with a creamy Caesar dressing. Also available without the chicken.

I ask the waitperson to leave off the croutons and substitute sweet garlic vinaigrette for the Caesar dressing.

Home Style Sides/Gourmet Sides:

Green Beans.

Garlicky Lemon Spinach.

Creamed Spinach.

Fresh Steamed Vegetables.

Market Pairs:

Chose two of your favorites to create a delicious combination.

Half Sandwich.

Half Salad.

Bowl of Soup.

Regular Side.

California Pastrami

Chain Restaurant

On all combination sandwiches I substitute the tossed salad for the side of French fries that comes with the sandwich. My husband and I share one sandwich. When he is not with me, I order the 1/2 size sandwich. We eat here on reward days.

Pastrami Sandwiches:

Classic California Pastrami.

Classic California Pastrami Combo.

1/2 Classic Combo

Eastern Style Pastrami Combo – With a pickle spear and a choice of potato salad or coleslaw. I order the coleslaw and ask the counter person to ask the chef to substitute the side salad for the French fries.

1/2 Eastern Style Pastrami - With a pickle spear and a choice of potato salad or coleslaw. I order the coleslaw and ask the counterperson to ask the chef to substitute the side salad for the French fries.

1/2 Eastern Style Pastrami Combo - With a pickle spear and a choice of potato salad or coleslaw. I order the coleslaw and ask the counterperson to ask the chef to substitute the side salad for the French fries.

Eastern Style Pastrami Alone – Without the side of pickle and without potato salad or coleslaw.

Eastern Style Pastrami Alone Combo – It comes with a drink and fries but without the side of pickle and without the potato salad or coleslaw.

Grilled Sandwiches:

Reuben.

Reuben Combo.

Reuben 1/2 Size.

Rueben 1/2 Size Combo.

Corned Beef – Fresh sliced steamed corned beef on rye bread grilled with Swiss cheese and Thousand Island Dressing. I ask the counterperson to ask the chef to substitute yellow mustard for the Thousand Island dressing.

Corned Beef Combo.

Corned Beef Alone.

Corned Beef Alone Combo.

Corned Beef 1/2 Size.

Corned Beef 1/2 Size Combo.

Corned Beef Mustard Only.

Corned Beef Mustard Only Combo.

Corned Beef Mustard only Alone Combo

Hot Sandwiches:

Rib Eye Steak Sandwich - Thin cut choice Rib Eye Steak, lightly seasoned & grilled to perfection served on a fresh Hoagie Roll w/mayonnaise, lettuce and tomato.

Rib Eye Steak Sandwich Combo.

Roast Beef – Fresh sliced Roast Beef simmered in Au Jus served on a fresh Hoagie Roll.

Roast Beef Combo

Veggie Sandwich

Veggie Sandwich Combo

Philly Cheese Steak – Thin cut choice steak with grilled onions, bell peppers, served on a fresh Hoagie Roll and topped with cheese.

Philly Cheese Steak Combo

Burgers:

Pastrami Burger.

Pastrami Burger Combo

Hamburger

Hamburger Combo

Cheeseburger

Cheeseburger Combo

Double Cheeseburger

Double Cheeseburger Combo.

Cold Sandwiches:

Turkey Sandwich – A triple decker sandwich with sliced turkey, Swiss cheese, and lettuce. I ask the counterperson to ask the chef to leave out the middle and top slice of bread and to serve it open faced.

Turkey Sandwich Combo

Dion's

Chain Restaurant

Subs:

Our submarines are made to order, served on toasted Original White or Wheat baguettes with your choice of side. Subs are customizable. 6 inch or 10 inch. Green Chile available upon request for an additional charge. Choose your side item. Fruit or koolslaw. I order the sub served open faced with coleslaw.

<u>Turkey & Swiss</u> - Sliced red onions, tomatoes, lettuce, mayonnaise & deli mustard. Served with side, pickle spear & Greek dressing.

<u>Pastrami & Provolone</u> – Sliced red onions, tomatoes, lettuce, mayonnaise & deli mustard. Served with side, pickle spear & Greek dressing.

<u>Roast Beef & Provolone</u> - Sliced red onions, tomatoes, lettuce, mayonnaise & deli mustard. Served with side, pickle spear & Greek dressing.

<u>Meatball & Provolone</u> – Served with a side and a cup of pizza sauce.

<u>Veggie (Green Chile & Cheddar)</u> – Sliced red onions, bell peppers, mushrooms, black olives, tomatoes, lettuce, mayonnaise & deli mustard. Served with side, pickle spear & Greek dressing. I ask the counterperson to ask the chef to substitute extra onions or bell peppers for the black olives.

Salads:

Healthy and delicious, our salads are made to order using fresh vegetables and crisp lettuce, with a side of dressing made from scratch. All salads are customizable. Available half, full, or family size. Substitute Romaine or spring mix lettuce for an additional charge. Dion's mix" is diced cucumbers, red onions & bell peppers.

Ranch Salad – Iceberg lettuce, pastrami, provolone, tomatoes, croutons & Dion's mix. I ask the counterperson to ask the chef to substitute extra lettuce for the croutons.

Chef Salad – Iceberg lettuce, ham, cheddar, sliced egg, tomatoes, croutons & Dion's mix. I ask the counterperson to ask the chef to substitute turkey for the ham and to leave off the croutons.

Greek Salad – Iceberg lettuce, black olives, feta, tomatoes, croutons & Dion's mix. I ask the counterperson to ask the chef to substitute extra lettuce for the black olives and croutons. For a variation, I order it with turkey.

Turkey Salad – Iceberg lettuce, turkey, provolone, tomatoes, croutons & Dion's mix. I ask the counterperson to ask the chef to substitute extra lettuce for the croutons.

Tossed Salads:

Half, full, or family size. Iceberg lettuce, tomatoes, croutons & Dion's mix. I ask the counterperson to ask the chef to substitute extra lettuce for the croutons.

Gourmet Salads:

Half, full, or family size.

Chicken Caesar – Romaine lettuce grilled chicken strips, croutons & shredded parmesan. I ask the counterperson to ask the chef to substitute extra lettuce for the croutons and to substitute bleu cheese dressing for the Caesar dressing.

Gourmet Chicken Salad – Spring mix lettuce, grilled chicken strips, pecans, bleu cheese crumbles & tomatoes.

Dion's Dressings (Homemade):

Ranch, Greek, Raspberry Vinaigrette, Bleu Cheese,

Extras:

Fresh seasonal fruit (cup), koolslaw (cup).

Five Guys® Burgers & Fries

Chain Restaurant

Burgers:

Hamburger.

Little Hamburger.

Sandwiches:

Veggie Sandwich.

Toppings:

All toppings are free. (Everything or all the way receives only toppings listed in black)

Mayo – (black).

Lettuce – (black).

Pickles – (black).

Tomatoes – (black).

Grilled Onions – (black).

Grilled Mushrooms – (black).

Mustard – (black).

Relish – (red).

Onions – (red).

Green Peppers – (red).

Flying Star Café

Chain Restaurant

Fresh Salads:

Flying Star salads feature humanely farmed chicken breasts cage free organic eggs, & homemade dressings: Ranch, Bleu Cheese, Spicy Asian Sesame, Tomatillo Lime Vinaigrette (house), and Thai Vinaigrette.

Indulge: Customize your salad by adding one of the following meat options for an extra charge: Grilled chicken breast or NM sirloin.

Crave – Bleu cheese, toasted almonds, field greens, fresh strawberries, tart apples, oranges & dried cranberries tossed in a Tomatillo Lime Vinaigrette. For an extra charge add a scoop of chicken salad or grilled chicken.

Chinese Crunch – Choice of grilled chicken or organic tofu with cool, crisp veggies tossed with Spicy Asian Sesame dressing, toasted almonds & crunchy wonton strips. I order the grilled chicken and ask the counterperson to ask the chef to substitute extra greens for the crunchy wonton strips.

Chicken Caesar – The classic topped with grilled chicken breast, our bakery croutons & shaved Romano. I ask the counterperson to ask the chef to substitute extra greens for the croutons and to substitute bleu cheese for the Caesar dressing.

Thai Steak Salad – New Mexico ranched sirloin steak strips top our chopped, 8 vegetable salad (too numerous to list) & kicks it up with fresh mint, cilantro & an eyes wide open dressing. Hidden beneath this cool, lean salad are whole wheat noodles tossed with peanut sauce. I ask the counterperson to ask the chef to substitute extra greens for the whole wheat noodles.

Greek Goddess – Big chunks of crispy batter dipped feta cheese atop chopped Romaine tossed in Avocado Vinaigrette.

Garnished with fresh avocado slices, olives, tomatoes, lemon wedges & basil. I ask the counter person to ask the chef to substitute extra tomatoes for the avocado slices and to substitute Tomatillo Lime Vinaigrette dressing for the Avocado Vinaigrette.

Chopped Cobb – The American favorite classically interpreted. House roasted turkey, Applewood smoked bacon, chopped hardboiled egg, bleu cheese avocado and tomato over crisp greens. Served with our Tomatillo Lime Vinaigrette. I ask the counterperson to ask the chef to substitute extra roasted turkey for the bacon and to substitute extra tomato for the avocado.

Lite Greens – A lovely salad perfect for a small meal. Choice of dressing.

Cup of Soup & Lite Greens – Check our specials board or ask a counter server for what's fresh today.

Sandwiches:

Choose fresh coleslaw or fresh fruit salad. I ask the counterperson to ask the chef to serve all sandwiches open faced.

Rancher's Melt – Our classic sandwich; thinly sliced lightly sautéed local sirloin, chopped green chile, tomato slices, horseradish sauce & Jack on thick slices of grilled sourdough.

Turkey Jack – (#1 favorite since 1988). House roasted turkey, New Mexico green chile, tomatoes & Jack on grilled sourdough.

Grilled Chicken Breast – Jack cheese, lettuce, tomatoes, red onion, pickles & Cajun dressing on our big hamburger bun.

Californian – (Since 1988) Marinated, grilled Crimini mushrooms, Swiss, avocado, tomatoes, caramelized onions & ranch dressing on grilled sourdough. I ask the counterperson to ask the chef to substitute extra tomatoes for the avocado.

Big Burgers:

Chose fresh coleslaw or fresh fruit salad.

NM Burger – Chopped green chile & melted cheddar.

Blues Burger – Bleu cheese crumbles, sizzled Applewood bacon & Swiss. I ask the counterperson to ask the chef to substitute extra Swiss for the Applewood bacon.

Hamburger Classic – Cheese is an extra charge.

Petite Burger

Chilly:

Chicken Salad – Poached chicken breast, dill, onion, mayo, lettuce & tomatoes.

Turkey Swiss – House roasted turkey breast, Swiss, fresh tomatoes, lettuce, mayo & mustard.

Dinner All Day:

Chicken Couscous – Light yet very satisfying – herbed, grilled chicken breast served over Israeli pearl couscous pilaf & steamed broccoli florets. Finished with a drizzle of extra virgin olive oil/white balsamic vinegar & feta crumbles. I ask the counterperson to ask the chef to substitute extra broccoli florets for the couscous.

Stew Pot Chicken – With a big country biscuit. Big chunks of white meat chicken breast, sweet potatoes, peas, Crimini mushrooms & zucchini stewed in light, deeply flavorful green chile gravy. I do not eat the biscuit.

New Mexico Chile Beef Stew – Hearty, spicy, red or green. Spiked with seasoned ground beef from local ranches & tasty pinto beans. Topped with cheddar Jack cheeses & diced tomatoes. Served with a big flour tortilla. I do not eat the tortilla.

Fuddruckers

Chain Restaurant

Specialty Burgers:

1/3 lb., 1/2 lb, 2/3lb., and 1lb.

Three Cheeses – Cheddar, Swiss, Monterey Jack Cheese.

Inferno – Spicy jalapenos, grilled onions, pepper Jack cheese.

Swiss Melt – Grilled mushrooms, grilled onions, Swiss cheese.

Exotics:

Buffalo

The Original World's Greatest Burger:

We cook it. You top it.

1/3lb., 1/2lb., 2/3lb., 1lb.

Grilled onions, choice of cheese, and grilled onions are an extra charge.

Chicken:

We cook it. You top it. Grilled chicken breast.

Customize your chicken with our specialty toppings.

Fudds Favs:

Turkey Burger.

Ribeye Steak Sandwich.

Salads:

All salads (except Taco Salad) include grilled or crispy chicken breast. I always order the grilled chicken breast.

Chicken Caesar – A traditional favorite with Caesar dressing & parmesan cheese. I ask the counter person to ask the chef to leave off the croutons and to substitute another dressing for the Caesar dressing.

Market Toss – Monterey Jack & cheddar cheeses, tomatoes, eggs, almonds & bacon. I ask the counter person to ask the chef to substitute extra tomatoes for the bacon.

Taco Salad – Grilled chicken or ground beef, cheddar, pico de Gallo, guacamole & sour cream, served in an edible shell. I ask the counter person to ask the chef to substitute tomatoes for the guacamole. I do not eat the shell.

Napa Valley – Romaine lettuce, bleu cheese, apples, dried cranberries & almonds.

Platters:

Chopped Steak – Served with grilled onions, mushrooms & a side salad.

Just For Kids:

For your kids or the grandkids. Includes a drink and choice of apple wedges, fruit cup or cole slaw. For kids 12 & under.

Hamburger.

Cheeseburger.

Sides:

Fruit Medley.

Coleslaw.

Condiments & Toppings:

Jalapeno Cheese Sauce.

Cheddar Cheese Sauce.

Mayonnaise.

Spicy Brown Mustard.

Yellow Mustard.

Tomato Salsa.

Sliced Tomatoes.

Sliced Jalapenos.

Pickle Slices.

Leaf Lettuce.

Shredded Lettuce.

Sliced White Onions.

Grand Traverse Pie Company

Chain Restaurant

Classic Sandwiches:

Turkey & Cheddar – Oven roasted turkey, tomatoes and lettuce with mayo served on sourdough.

Mediterranean Veggie – Roasted red pepper, red onion, cucumber, tomato, feta cheese, lettuce and salt and pepper on an herbed baguette. I ask the counterperson to ask the chef to substitute extra roasted red pepper for the cucumber.

Specialty Sandwiches:

Chicken Pesto with Roasted Red Pepper – Baked chicken breast, roasted red pepper, lettuce with pesto mayo on focaccia.

Herbed Italian – Smoked ham, pepperoncini, tomatoes, roasted red peppers, red onion, pepperoni, lettuce & Med. Feta dressing on herbed baguette. I ask the counterperson to ask the chef to substitute turkey for the ham and pepperoni.

GT Chicken Salad – Fresh chicken salad mixed with grapes and dired cherries with lettuce and salt and pepper on a flakey croissant.

Caprese – Pesto mayo, fresh sliced mozzarella, tomatoes, baby spinach leaves, balsamic vinaigrette served on focaccia bread.

Specialty Grilled Sandwiches:

All sandwiches include one of our sides of: apple or coleslaw and a pickle.

Reuben on Rye – Thinly sliced corned beef, Swiss cheese, sauerkraut, 1000 Island Dressing on marble rye. I ask the counterperson to ask the chef to substitute mustard for the 1000 Island Dressing.

Turkey Reuben on Rye - Thinly sliced turkey, Swiss cheese, sauerkraut, 1000 Island Dressing on marble rye. I ask the counterperson to ask the chef to substitute mustard for the 1000 Island Dressing.

<u>Lighthouse Turkey Cheddar</u> – Turkey, cheddar cheese, tomato, salt and pepper with pesto mayo on whole wheat.

<u>Chicken Focaccia</u> – Baked chicken breast, Cherrywood smoked bacon, Swiss cheese and ranch served on focaccia. I ask the counterperson to ask the chef to substitute lettuce and tomato for the bacon.

<u>French Dip</u> – Oven roasted Angus beef, grilled red onions and Swiss cheese on a herbed baguette and served with warm au jus.

Comfort Foods:

<u>Chicken Pot Pie</u> – in our famous flaky crust – diced chicken, carrots, peas, lima beans, corn and green beans. I eat this pie on a reward day.

<u>Prime Rib Pot Pie</u> - in our famous flaky crust – prime rib, carrots, peas, lima beans, corn and green beans. I eat this pie on a reward day.

<u>Broccoli Cheddar Quiche</u>

<u>Spinach Mushroom Quiche</u>

<u>Chicken Quesadilla</u> – Baked chicken breast, tomatoes and cheddar with salsa ranch and grilled on a tomato wrap. I ask the counterperson to ask the chef to serve the quesadilla open faced.

Soups:

Soup of the day or one of our daily varieties.

Classic Salads:

<u>House Salad</u> – Bib lettuce blend, tomato, cucumber, red onion, feta cheese, parmesan cheese and croutons. I ask the counterperson to ask the chef to substitute extra lettuce and tomato for the cucumbers and croutons.

Greek Salad – Tomato, cucumber, red onion and crisp romaine lettuce tossed in feta dressing topped with feta cheese, kalamata olives and pepperoncini. I ask the counterperson to ask the chef to substitute extra romaine lettuce for the cucumbers.

Specialty Salads:

Add hot baked chicken to any salad for an additional charge.

Cherry Chicken Salad – Bib lettuce blend, hot baked chicken breast, tomato, cucumber, feta cheese, parmesan cheese, dried cherries and garlic croutons. I ask the waitperson to ask the chef to substitute extra lettuce and tomatoes for the cucumbers and croutons.

Fresh Pear Chicken Salad – Bib lettuce blend, fresh pears, hot baked chicken breast, bleu cheese, toasted pecans, garlic croutons and our own berry cherry vinaigrette. I ask the counterperson to ask the chef to substitute extra lettuce for the croutons.

Strawberry Fields Salad – Bib lettuce blend, fresh apples, mandarin oranges, fresh strawberries, red onion, toasted pecans and parmesan cheese.

Spinach Salad with Goat Cheese – Fresh baby spinach topped with blueberries, diced apples, sliced red onions, pecan pieces and goat cheese served with a side of honey-mustard vinaigrette.

Dressings:

House-made Ranch.

Chipotle Ranch.

Bleu Cheese.

Honey-Mustard Vinaigrette.

Honey-Mustard.

Balsamic Vinaigrette.

Mediterranean Feta.

Berry Cherry Vinaigrette.

Pies:

Chocolate Cream.

Coconut Cream.

Strawberry Peach.

Strawberry Rhubarb.

Cakes:

Carrot Cake.

Death by Chocolate.

Whole Hog Café

Chain Restaurant

Sandwiches:

All sandwiches are garnished with coleslaw. All meats dry rubbed with spices and smoked with pecan wood. Available regular or jumbo size.

Beef Brisket.

Pulled Chicken.

Plates:

Includes meat, 2 side orders and a dinner roll.

Beef Brisket.

Pulled Chicken.

Half Chicken – Served with skin on it. I remove the skin.

Salads:

Choice of Hidden Valley packaged dressing: Ranch, Italian, Blue Cheese, Honey Mustard, or Fat Free Raspberry Vinaigrette.

Salad – Iceberg/Romaine Lettuce.

Barbecue Salad -

Pulled Chicken.

Beef.

Side Orders:

Coleslaw.

Salad.

Jason's Deli

Chain Restaurant

Soups:

French Onion – I ask the counterperson to ask the chef to leave out the bread and croutons.

Organic Vegetable

Tomato Basil

Broccoli Cheese

Salads:

Available in original or lighter portion. If I am eating the salad as a meal, I order the original size.

The Big Chef- Ham, turkey breast, Swiss, cheddar, tomatoes, kalamata olives, hard-boiled egg slices on mixed greens. I ask the counterperson to ask the chef to substitute extra turkey breast for the ham.

Nutty Mixed-Up Salad – Natural, grilled chicken breast, organic field greens, grapes, feta, nuts, dried cranberries, raisins, pumpkin seeds, organic apples. I ask the counterperson to ask the chef to substitute extra organic field greens for the grapes and pumpkin seeds.

Chicken Club Salad – Natural, grilled chicken breast, grape tomatoes, sliced avocado, cheddar, asiago, bacon on mixed salad greens. I ask the counterperson to ask the chef to substitute extra grape tomatoes for the avocado and bacon.

Chicken Caesar – Natural, grilled chicken breast, romaine, asiago, croutons, creamy Caesar dressing. I ask the waitperson to ask the chef to substitute bleu cheese dressing for the Caesar dressing and to leave off the croutons.

Meatless Eats:

Garden Fresh Salad Bar – Indulge all you like! Fresh organics, dozens of toppings, real cheeses, fresh-made sides and famous mini-muffins. I do not eat the muffins, bacon bits, pumpkin seeds, avocado, or croutons.

Add a side of: chicken salad with almonds and pineapple, turkey, smoked turkey, or natural grilled chicken breast for an additional charge.

Zucchini Grillini - Grilled zucchini, Muenster, organic spinach, red onions, Roma tomatoes, kalamata olives, roasted red pepper, hummus, toasted on 9-grain artisan bread. Served with fresh fruit, steamed veggies, or baked chips. I order the fresh fruit or steamed veggies. I ask the counterperson to ask the chef to substitute extra spinach and red onions for the hummus and toasted 9-grain artisan bread.

Build Your Own Veggie Sandwich - Your choice of bread, cheese, spreads and toppings! Served with chips or baked chips. I ask the counterperson to ask the chef to substitute extra veggies for the chips.

Fresh Fruit Plate - Served with creamy fruit dip.

Fresh Fruit Cup – Served with creamy fruit dip.

Side Salad or Caesar Side Salad – Available for an extra charge with an entrée purchase. On the Caesar salad I ask the counterperson to ask the chef to substitute bleu cheese dressing for the Caesar dressing.

Specialty Sandwiches:

Served with chips or baked chips unless otherwise stated. I ask the counterperson to ask the chef to substitute extra vegetables for the chips.

Amy's Turkey-O – Toasted onion bun with turkey breast, sliced avocado, jalapeno pepper Jack, red onions, Roma tomatoes, lettuce and stone ground mustard. I ask the counterperson to ask the chef to substitute extra tomatoes for the avocado.

Santa Fe Chicken Sandwich® - Natural, grilled chicken breast, bacon, Swiss, guacamole, tomato, Russian dressing, grilled on whole grain wheat. I ask the counterperson to ask the chef to substitute lettuce for the guacamole and extra Swiss for the bacon.

The Papa Joe – Named for our Founder's Dad. Toasted herb focaccia with turkey breast, asiago, roasted tomatoes, walnut pesto, mayo.

Famous Favorites:

Served with chips or baked chips unless otherwise stated. I ask the counterperson to ask the chef to substitute extra vegetables for the chips.

Reuben The Great – 1/2 pound of hot corned beef or pastrami, Swiss, sauerkraut, Russian dressing, grilled on rye. I ask the counterperson to ask the chef to substitute yellow mustard for the Russian dressing.

The New York Yankee – 3/4 pound combo of hot corned beef and pastrami, Swiss and your choice of mustard or mayo, on rye.

Hot Corned Beef or Hot Pastrami Sandwich – 1/2 pound of hot corned beef or pastrami. Your choice of bread topped the way you like it.

Beefeater – 1/2 pound of hot roast beef, provolone, mayo on New Orleans French bread with a cup of au jus.

Build Your Own Sandwich:

Served with chips or baked chips. For an additional charge you can substitute fresh fruit for the chips.

Pick your meat, name your bread, select your spreads and dress it up. You also decide the size.

Oven-Roasted Turkey Breast

Smoked Turkey Breast

Roast Beef

Chicken Salad with almonds and pineapple

Telera Bread

Whole Grain Wheat

White

Rye

9-Grain Artisan Bread

Herb Focaccia

All-Butter Croissant

Onion Bun

New Orleans French Bread

Gluten-Free Bread an extra charge.

Cheese an extra charge.

McAllister's Deli

Chain Restaurant

Starters:

Cup of Soup or Chili – (Traditional or Veggie).

Bowl of Soup or Chili – (Traditional or Veggie).

Chili Cheese Dip – (Traditional or Veggie) – Chili, Ro-tel® cheese dip, sliced jalapenos and tortilla chips. I do not eat the tortilla chips.

Entrée Salads:

Italian Chopped Salad – Black Forest ham, salami, olive salad, roasted red peppers, provolone, red onions, cucumbers, and tomatoes. Chef's dressing selection: Olive Oil & Balsamic Vinaigrette. I ask the counter person to ask the chef to substitute turkey for the ham and extra tomatoes for the cucumbers.

Grilled Chicken Salad – Grilled chicken breast, Applewood smoked bacon, cheddar – Jack cheese, tomatoes, cucumbers and croutons. I ask the waitperson to ask the chef to substitute extra cheddar for the bacon and extra greens for the cucumbers and croutons.

Chef Salad – Black Forest ham, Butterball™ smoked turkey, Applewood smoked bacon, cheddar – Jack cheese, tomatoes, cucumbers and croutons. I ask the waitperson to ask the chef to substitute extra turkey for the ham and bacon and to substitute extra greens for the cucumbers and croutons.

Grilled Chicken Caesar – Grilled chicken breast, Romaine, Parmesan and croutons, tossed with Caesar dressing. I ask the waitperson to ask the chef to substitute extra Romaine for the croutons and to substitute bleu cheese dressing for the Caesar dressing.

Savannah Chopped Salad - Grilled chicken breast, dried cranberries, gorgonzola cheese, honey roasted almonds, tomatoes and cucumbers. Chef's dressing selection: Sherry Shallot. I ask the waitperson to ask the chef to substitute extra tomatoes for the cucumbers.

Garden Salad – Fresh greens, cheddar – Jack cheese, tomatoes, cucumbers and croutons. I ask the waitperson to ask the chef to substitute extra greens for the cucumbers and croutons.

With a scoop of harvest chicken salad for an extra charge.

Dressings – McAlister's Honey Mustard™, Ranch, Olive Oil & Balsamic Vinaigrette, Bleu Cheese, Parmesan Peppercorn, and Sherry Shallot.

Hot Sandwiches:

Served with a pickle and choice of side.

French Dip – A quarter pound of USDA choice Black Angus roast beef and sharp cheddar on a baguette, served au jus.

Reuben – Corned beef, sauerkraut, Swiss and Thousand Island dressing on toasted rye bread. I ask the waitperson to ask the chef to substitute mustard for the Thousand Island dressing.

Melts – Turkey or Roast Beef. Butterball™ smoked turkey or USDA choice Black Angus roast beef, sharp cheddar, Applewood smoked bacon, lettuce, tomatoes, spicy brown mustard, lite mayo on a toasted 6" wheat hoagie. I ask the counterperson to ask the chef to substitute extra tomatoes for the bacon.

Southwest Turkey Melt – Butterball™ smoked turkey, Applewood smoked bacon, pepper jack cheese, spicy guacamole and Chipotle Ranch. Topped with lettuce and tomatoes on a baguette. I ask the counterperson to ask the chef to substitute extra turkey for the bacon and extra tomatoes for the guacamole.

The New Yorker™ - Corned beef, pastrami, Swiss and spicy brown mustard on toasted rye bread.

Memphian™ - USDA choice Black Angus roast beef, Black Forest ham, Butterball™ smoked turkey, provolone, lettuce, tomatoes, lite mayo and spicy brown mustard on a toasted 6" wheat hoagie. I ask the counterperson to ask the chef to substitute extra turkey for the ham.

The Big Nasty ® - Over a third of a pound of tender, USDA choice Black Angus roast beef served open-faced on a toasted baguette with gravy and cheddar-Jack cheese. I ask the counterperson to ask the chef to leave off the gravy.

Choose 2 – Cup of soup with half of any salad or sandwich, or two half portions of any salad or sandwich.

Classic Sandwiches:

Served with a pickle and a choice of side.

Italian Submarine – Black Forest ham, salami, Swiss, lettuce, tomatoes, red onions, bell peppers and black olives, topped with olive oil and vinegar, salt, pepper and spicy brown mustard on a toasted baguette. I ask the counter person to ask the chef to substitute turkey for the ham and to leave off the salt.

Harvest Chicken Salad – Dressed with leaf lettuce and tomatoes on a toasted croissant

Grilled Chicken – Grilled chicken breast, lettuce tomatoes, Swiss and McAllister's Honey Mustard™ on a toasted croissant.

Deli Classics – Turkey, Roast Beef, Corned Beef, Pastrami or Salami served on your choice of bread, dressed with lettuce, tomatoes and spicy brown mustard. You can add cheese for an additional charge

Sides:

Coleslaw.

Fruit Cup.

Steamed Veggies.

Substitute a cup of soup or a side salad for an additional charge.

Desserts:

Chocolate Lovin' Spooncake.

Colossal Carrot Cake.

Brownies.

Newk's® Express Café

Chain Restaurant

Fresh Tossed Salads:

Visit Newk's roundtable for breadsticks and toppings.

Newk's Favorite – Mixed greens, grilled chicken breast, gorgonzola cheese, dried cranberries, grapes, artichoke hearts, pecans and croutons tossed with Newk's sherry vinaigrette. I ask the counterperson to ask the chef to substitute extra dried cranberries for the grapes and croutons.

Ultimate – Mixed greens, grilled chicken breast, ham, turkey, bacon, grape tomatoes, cucumbers, cheddar cheese and croutons tossed with Newk's original honey mustard dressing. I ask the counterperson to ask the chef to substitute extra turkey for the ham and bacon and to substitute extra tomatoes for the cucumbers and croutons.

Black & Bleu – Mixed greens, choice beef tender, gorgonzola cheese, pecans, grape tomatoes, and sliced red onion tossed with bleu cheese dressing.

Cobb – Mixed greens, grilled chicken breast, bacon, eggs, gorgonzola cheese, grape tomatoes, green onions, pecans and croutons tossed with bleu cheese dressing. I ask the counterperson to ask the chef to substitute extra grape tomatoes and green onions for the bacon and the croutons.

Chef – Mixed greens, ham, turkey, grape tomatoes, cucumbers, cheddar cheese and croutons tossed with your choice of dressing. I ask the counterperson to ask the chef to substitute extra turkey for the ham and extra grape tomatoes for the cucumbers and croutons.

Southern – Mixed greens, a scoop of Newk's homemade chicken salad, grape tomatoes, and croutons. I ask the counterperson to ask the chef to leave off the croutons.

Greek – Romaine, feta cheese, kalamata olives, grape tomatoes, artichoke hearts, cucumbers, pepperoncini peppers and sliced red onion tossed with Newk's Greek dressing. I ask the counterperson to ask the chef to substitute extra grape tomatoes for the cucumbers.

Simply Half – Mixed greens, grape tomatoes, cucumbers, carrots, cheddar cheese and croutons with your favorite dressing. Also available as a whole salad. I ask the counterperson to ask the chef to substitute extra grape tomatoes for the cucumbers and croutons.

Salad Dressings:

Newk's original honey mustard.

Ranch.

Balsamic Vinaigrette.

Greek.

Bleu Cheese.

Sherry Vinaigrette.

Remoulade.

Soup of the Day:

Available in small – 8 oz., large – 16 oz., or jumbo – 32 oz.

Combos:

Half a sandwich and half a salad. (Simply or Caesar Salad). On the Caesar salad I ask the counterperson to ask the chef to leave off the croutons and to substitute bleu cheese dressing for the Caesar dressing.

Bowl of soup and half a salad. On the Caesar salad I ask the counterperson to ask the chef to leave off the croutons and to substitute bleu cheese dressing for the Caesar dressing.

Half a sandwich and a cup of soup.

Toasted Sandwiches:

All sandwiches are made to order and served warm on a fresh roll dressed with Hellmann's mayo, spicy Creole mustard, romaine lettuce, and tomato. If requested, we will add: Newk's original honey mustard, onion, pickle, Italian sauce.

Chicken Salad – Homemade with grapes, pecans with provolone cheese.

Roast Beef – with provolone cheese.

Turkey Breast – Oven roasted with Swiss cheese.

Toasted Specialty Sandwiches:

All sandwiches served with your choice of coleslaw or fresh fruit.

Pesto Chicken – Grilled chicken breast, pesto, roasted red and yellow bell peppers and goat cheese.

Grilled Steak – Choice beef tender, marinated and grilled, sliced thin, layered with caramelized onions, provolone cheese and horseradish spread.

Italian – Capicola, mortadella, pepperoni, salami, provolone cheese, mayo, spicy Creole mustard, lettuce, tomato, yellow onions, hot cherry peppers and Italian sauce. I ask the counterperson to ask the chef to substitute extra lettuce and tomato for the capicola and mortadella and to leave off the hot cherry peppers.

Grilled Chicken – Grilled chicken breast, olive oil, Applewood smoked bacon, Swiss cheese, lettuce, tomato, mayo and Newk's original honey mustard. I ask the counterperson to ask the chef to substitute extra Swiss cheese for the Applewood smoked bacon.

Royal – Salami, ham, turkey, roast beef, Swiss cheese, mayo, spicy Creole mustard, lettuce and tomato. I ask the counterperson to ask the chef to substitute extra roast beef for the ham.

Newk's "Q" – Newk's white BBQ sauce, grilled chicken breast,

Applewood smoked bacon, and white cheddar cheese with tomato. I ask the counterperson to ask the chef to substitute extra white cheddar cheese for the Applewood smoked bacon.

Paradise Bakery & Café/Panera/St. Louis Bread Company

Chain Restaurant

Paradise Bakery & Café's menu is not listed here because in the first edition of *FROM FAT TO FABULOUS: A DIET GUIDE FOR RESTAURANT LOVERS,* it is listed under St. Louis Bread Company/Panera Bread.

Building on the success of its Panera Cares program that allows diners to pay what they can for a meal, in select locations the company is now offering select meals at no set price. Diners can either pay the suggested price, pay more to cover the cost of someone else's meal, or pay what they can.

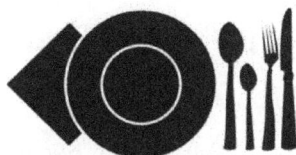

SUPERMARKET PREPARED FOODS

BREAKFAST/LUNCH/DINER

Albertsons

Supermarket Chain

Deli Counter:

Baked Chicken.

Rotisserie Chicken.

Waldorf Salad.

Smoked or Oven Browned Turkey Breast.

Rotisserie Turkey Breast.

Mozzarella and Tomato Salad.

Swiss, Provolone, or Munster Cheese.

Fresh Made Party Trays:

The Crowd Pleaser – Roast beef, premium turkey breast, baked ham, domestic Swiss cheese, Provolone and sliced American cheese plus our all-American potato salad. I ask the counterperson to ask the chef to substitute extra turkey breast for the ham, extra Swiss for the American cheese, and coleslaw for the potato salad.

Gourmet Meat Tray – A delicious selection of sliced meats that includes smoked turkey breast, baked ham, roast beef, and premium turkey breast garnished with olives and sweet baby gherkins. I ask the counterperson to ask the chef to substitute extra roast beef for the ham and sour pickles for the sweet baby gherkins.

"Cheese Please" Party Tray – Cheese to please, a cornucopia of imported and domestic cheeses. Edam, Swiss, American, Munster, Cheddar, hot pepper Jack, smoked Cheddar, blue cheese, and Gouda. I ask the counterperson to ask the chef to substitute extra cheddar cheese for the American cheese.

Fresh Fruit & Cheese Tray – Rich, tasty Cheddar, Havarti, and domestic Swiss cheese with refreshing strawberries, grapes, cantaloupe and pineapple. (Fruits may vary by season.) I ask the counterperson to ask the chef to substitute extra pineapple and strawberries for the grapes and cantaloupe.

Salad Tray – Seven tempting salads on one platter. Pick and choose your favorites.

Fresh Vegetable Tray – Eating healthy never tasted so good. A harvest of fresh, crisp garden vegetables with our delicious ranch dip. Mushrooms, baby carrots, celery, broccoli, zucchini, and tomatoes.

Fresh Cut Vegetable Tray – Ready to serve fresh vegetable tray with ranch dip. Or select a fresh produce tray, both available in the produce department.

Fresh Cut Fruit Tray – Fresh medley of assorted fruit cut fresh.

Deviled Egg Tray – A holiday favorite that guests of all ages will enjoy. 24 generously filled half eggs. Fresh and ready to go in the produce department.

Dierbergs' Kitchens

Supermarket Chain

Breakfast:

Low Carb Crustless Florentine Quiche.

Low Carb Crustless Vegetable Quiche.

Roasted Vegetable & Swiss Gruyere Frittata – I eat 1/4th of it.

Mushroom Florentine Gruyere Frittata – I eat 1/4th of it.

Fresh Strawberries.

Bigelow decaffeinated or herb tea.

Lunch/Dinner:

Flame Grilled Fresh Asparagus.

Cranberry Walnut Fresh Green Salad.

Broccoli, Cauliflower & Carrot Medley.

Fresh Vegetable Medley.

Roasted Brussels Sprouts.

Herb Green Bean Amandine.

Savory Carrots and Sugar Snap Peas.

Grilled Chicken Breasts.

Roasted Chicken – whole.

Roasted Chicken – pulled.

Deluxe Whole Roasted Turkey.

Succulent Prime Rib – with demi-glace and creamy horseradish sauces.

House-Made Beef Brisket – I ask the deli counterperson to slice it for me.

I do not eat the sauce that comes in the pre-sliced packages.

Slow Roasted Beef Brisket Au Jus.

Meat Loaf with tomato sauce – Because it has bread crumbs in it, I only eat it on a reward day.

Meatballs – Because they have bread crumbs in them, I only eat them on a reward day.

Parmesan Encrusted Chicken.

From the salad bar – iceberg lettuce, Romaine lettuce, tomatoes, onions, mushrooms, green peppers.

Dierbergs' Ultimate Party Guide:

Garden Classics Salad Bar:

Vegetable Garden Appetizer Platter – A hearty helping of delicious vegetable dip wets the appetite in this taste-tempting platter loaded with garden-fresh vegetables. Baby carrots, cucumbers, broccoli, cauliflower, grape tomatoes, and broccoli. I ask the deli counterperson to substitute extra tomatoes for the cucumbers.

Festive Luau Bowls – These bountiful, deep-dish luau bowls, filled with fresh seasonal fruit or garden vegetable cutlets compliment any occasion. Produce varies by season. The fruit bowl contains blue berries, strawberries, pineapple, and green and pink melons. I ask the deli counterperson to substitute extra fruit for the melons. The vegetable bowl contains the same vegetables as the Vegetable Garden Appetizer Platter.

Watermelon Boat – contains the same fruits as the Festive Luau Bowl.

Italian Salad – Enjoy a Se. Louis favorite tossed fresh with chopped iceberg and romaine lettuce, artichoke hearts, red onions, peppers, parmesan cheese and Dierbergs' house dressing.

Caesar Salad – This salad classic combines fresh romaine lettuce with grated parmesan cheese, Diergbergs' homemade croutons and our special Caesar dressing. Also available with grilled chicken. I ask the deli counterperson to leave off the croutons and to substitute Italian or bleu cheese dressing for the Caesar dressing.

Zia's Italian Salad – Zia's signature sweet Italian dressing tops freshly chopped iceberg and romaine lettuce, grated parmesan cheese, peppers, and creamy provel cheese.

Party Classics Deli:

Carved Watermelon Fruit & Cheese Medley – A rainbow of fresh fruit cascades from a carved watermelon complemented with fancy cut, natural cheese cubes. Strawberries, pineapples, watermelon, and grapes. I ask the deli counterperson to substitute extra fruit for the grapes.

Cheese Snacker's Favorite – Fancy crackers and fresh fruit complement a platter loaded with Wisconsin cheeses: Muenster, Colby, marbled Jackby, Swiss, Swiss & rye, and salami cheese. I ask the deli counterperson to substitute extra strawberries for the grapes.

Gourmet Cheese & Fruit Kabobs – Our stunning pineapple fruit kabob tree is surrounded with an assortment of grapes, fruit dip and cheeses, including French Brie, French Boursin, Danish Havarti, Holland Smoked Gouda, and baby Gouda wedges. I ask the deli counterperson to substitute extra strawberries for the grapes.

Simple Elegance Deli:

Brie & Gorgonzola Torte – layers of luscious creamy Brie and Gorgonzola cheese spreads are encased with crushed walnuts and lovely garnishes for a first-class appetizer.

International Cheese Platter – A taste exploration, featuring classic cheeses from around the world, including Danish Havarti, French Brie, French Boursin, Norwegian Jarlsberg, creamy Danish blue, baby Gouda, and Italian-style Asiago. I ask the deli counterperson to substitute strawberries for the grapes.

Sandwich Essentials Deli:

Wafer Meat & Cheese Tray – lean, cooked deli ham, top-round roast beef, and smoked or regular turkey breast are wafer sliced and mounted on a tiered platter with American and Lorraine Swiss cheeses. I ask the deli counterperson to substitute extra turkey for the ham and extra Swiss cheese for the American cheese.

Chilled Beef Tenderloin Platter – Herbs and cracked peppercorns encrust Dierbergs' choice beef tenderloin – roasted, chilled, and sliced into medallions. Served with honey Dijon, creamy horseradish, and sherry-peppercorn sauces.

Gourmet Meat Platter – Our finest selection of sliced meats, including lean top-round roast beef, honey-mesquite turkey breast and our naturally smoked, honey-cured or Virginia-style ham are folded and arranged by hand to create a magnificent presentation. I ask the deli counterperson to substitute extra turkey for the ham.

Gourmet Meat & Cheese Tray – Top-round roast beef, honey-mesquite turkey, and naturally smoked ham are hand-placed with natural Wisconsin cheeses on this platter of gourmet sandwich essentials. I ask the deli counterperson to substitute extra turkey for the ham.

Sliced Variety Cheese Medley – Complement a meat platter with this lovely selection of Wisconsin Grade-A Swiss, Colby, marbled Jackby, and American cheeses. I ask the deli counterperson to substitute extra Swiss for the American cheese and to substitute strawberries for the grapes.

The Complete Sandwich Deli:

I do not eat deli sandwiches so only the sides are listed here.

Chilled Flame-Roasted Veggies – Fresh vegetables, roasted over an open-flame and tossed in a balsamic vinaigrette, offer exciting color, intense flavor, and delightful textures. Asparagus. mushrooms, zucchini, red and green peppers, and squash.

Casual Fare Deli:

Dierbergs' Barbecue and Grilled Favorites – Grilled chicken breasts and barbecued beef brisket. I ask the deli counterperson to slice fresh brisket without the sauce.

Schnucks

Party Guide
Chain Supermarket

Specialty Cheese Platters:

Connoisseur's Selection – Decorated Brie with Mascarpone, apricot preserves and encrusted with slivered almonds, Danish blue cheese, Danish fontina cheese, Boursin, Black Diamond cheddar, double Gloucester Stilton, goat cheese, and Saga blue cheese with grapes and strawberries. I ask the deli counterperson to substitute extra cheese for the apricot preserves and grapes.

Three Cheese Course – Hoop Cheddar, Jarlsberg, Havarti, Brie, smoked Gouda, extra sharp cheddar, and Danish blue cheese with grapes and strawberries. I ask the deli counterperson to substitute extra strawberries for the grapes.

Fresh Fruit Splendor – Pineapple chunks, strawberries, grapes, watermelon, kiwi, honeydew and cantaloupe served with a tasty fruit dip. I ask the counter person to substitute extra strawberries for the grapes.

Garden Delight – Grape tomatoes, radishes, celery sticks, baby style carrots, green onions, black pitted olives, Spanish stuffed green olives, sweet midgets and baby dill pickles. I ask the waitperson to substitute extra tomatoes for the sweet midgets.

Fruit & Cheese Delight – Fresh pineapple chunks, red seedless grapes, honeydew, strawberries, longhorn Colby cheese, Havarti cheese, and smoked Gouda cheese served with a tasty fruit dip. I ask the deli counterperson to substitute extra strawberries for the grapes.

Watermelon Basket – Hand-carved melon basket filled with watermelon, cantaloupe, pineapple, honeydew, blueberries, strawberries, and grapes. I ask the deli counterperson to substitute strawberries for the grapes.

Fresh Garden Vegetables & Dip – A selection of six dipping vegetables; cucumber slices, baby style carrots, celery sticks, broccoli, cauliflower, and grape tomatoes with your choice of onion or dill dip. I order the onion dip and ask the deli counterperson to substitute extra tomatoes for the cucumber slices.

Condiment Platter – Leaf lettuce, sliced pickles, shredded lettuce, green pepper, tomato, pepperoncini, and red onion with sub dressing, mayonnaise and honey mustard.

Holiday Delights!:

Cheese Appetizer – Colby Jack, longhorn Colby, Swiss, supers sharp and pepper Jack cheese cubes served with fruit garnish. I ask the deli counterperson to substitute strawberries for the grapes.

Party Pleaser – Roll-ups layered with roast beef and Colby Jack cheese, smoked turkey and longhorn Colby cheese, ham and baby Swiss cheese, hard salami and provolone cheese wedges, and super sharp and pepper Jack cheese cubes. I ask the deli counterperson to substitute extra roast beef and turkey for the ham and hard salami.

Meat and Cheese Roll-Ups – Roll-ups layered with roast beef and longhorn Colby cheese, turkey breast and Colby Jack cheese, ham and baby Swiss cheese, and hard salami with herb garlic cheese spread with hard-boiled eggs. I ask the deli counterperson to substitute extra roast beef and turkey for the ham and hard salami.

Gourmet Choice with Cheese – Roast beef, ham, and turkey breast with baby Swiss cheese and longhorn Colby cheese served with honey mustard. Customize your meats by choosing honey, smoked or natural flavor from our extensive collection. I ask the deli counterperson to substitute extra turkey for the ham.

Wafer Meat & Cheese – Wafer-sliced roast beef, turkey breast, and cooked ham, hard salami, baby Swiss, Colby Jack and yellow American cheese. I ask the deli counterperson to substitute extra turkey and roast beef for the ham and hard salami. I also ask that the extra Colby or Swiss cheese be substituted for the American cheese.

Cheese Lovers – Colby Jack, baby Swiss, hot pepper, Yellow American, sandwich-cut Swiss and longhorn Colby cheese garnished with fruit. I ask the deli counterperson to substitute extra Colby Jack for the American cheese and to substitute strawberries for the grapes.

Kitchen Fresh!:

Whether you need help with a holiday meal or a family dinner, let us do the cooking! You'll find only the best and freshest dishes from our Kitchen – fresh in-store within 24 hours! Our talented chefs, with years of culinary experience, use only the finest ingredients to create delicious entrées, salads and side dishes. You'll find a full selection of items like white meat chicken salad, meatloaf or broccoli raisin salad available every day in our Deli Department.

The Shnucks Difference!

Our Service Meat Department offers only the highest quality meats including top quality Certified Angus Beef®, fresh Perdue Poultry on ice, savory lamb, tender veal, and more. Choose our Schnucks Smokehouse smoked turkeys that you simply heat, serve, and enjoy! Order smoked turkeys three days in advance.

Smith's/Kroger's

Chain Supermarket

Deli Counter:

Papa John's Spanakopita Spinach Casserole – A spinach and feta cheese casserole. Papa John's does not sell it in their fast food establishments. The only place you can purchase it is at a supermarket deli counter.

Roasted Chicken – Available in parts or by the whole chicken. I remove the skin.

Innquasian Cusine Black Pepper Chicken – Boneless breast of chicken chunks, green beans, water chestnuts, red peppers, and onions in a brown sauce.

Party Platters:

Custom-made for you!

Luncheon Fare Deli Meat & Cheese:

Cubed Meat & Cheese – Bite-sized cubes of turkey, ham, Swiss and cheddar. I ask the counterperson to ask the chef to substitute extra turkey for the ham.

Deli Meat & Cheese – Our most popular deli meats and cheeses: premium Private Selection Oven Roasted Turkey, Smokehouse Ham, roast beef and more. I ask the counterperson to ask the chef to substitute extra roast beef for the ham.

Condiments – The ideal complement to our meat and cheese platters – and great for backyard barbecues too! Tomatoes, green peppers, red onions, shredded lettuce, pickles, and jalapenos.

Specialty Cheese & Fruit Platter – Our finest cheeses. Paired with grapes and assorted dried fruit. Including Brie, Stilton, Gruyere, Gouda and Parmigiano Reggiano. I ask the counterperson to substitute strawberries for the grapes.

Mouth-Watering Chicken & Ribs:

Baked Chicken – Seasoned and baked to perfection for juicy, delidious flavor in every bite. I cut off the skin.

Holiday Meals:

Roasted Turkey - perfectly roasted for tender, juicy taste in every bite. Fully cooked. Just heat in the oven and serve with your favorite side dishes.

Smoked Turkey – Cooked to perfection with a delicate, smoky flavor. Fully cooked. Just heat in the oven and serve with your favorite side dishes.

Prime Rib – Angus Choice, seasoned and slow-roasted for supreme tenderness. Fully cooked. Just heat in the oven and serve with your favorite side dishes.

Salads:

Flavorful combinations.

Tomato Mozzarella Balsamic – This delicious salad is made from fresh mozzarella, grape tomatoes, artichoke hearts and black olives tossed in white balsamic vinaigrette.

Broccoli Raisin – A crowd favorite that is rich in flavor. Broccoli, cauliflower, raisins, bacon and sunflower seeds are mixed together in a sweet and tangy dressing with a hint of lemon. I ask the counterperson to ask the chef to substitute extra broccoli for the bacon.

Spring Salad – Garnished with grape tomatoes, hard-boiled eggs, cucumber slices and your choice of dressing. I ask the counterperson to ask the chef to substitute extra grape tomatoes for the cucumbers.

Fruits & Vegetables:

Fresh & crisp.

Fresh Vegetable Platter – Crisp, crunchy veggies with plenty of creamy ranch for dipping. Organic varieties available in select locations. Carrots, Celery, radishes, broccoli, cauliflower, celery, green peppers, and cucumber slices.

Mozzarella Tomato – This simple salad will wow your guests. Made with fresh tomato slices, sliced mozzarella and basil. Available seasonally.

Sprouts Farmers Market

Country Kitchen
Chain Supermarket

Party Trays:

Spinach Dip – Dip on in for wonderful spinach goodness in every bite! Served with plenty of baguette slices.

Veggies – Crispy crunchy bites of healthy snacks. Garden-fresh seasonal vegetables with your choice of dip, creamy ranch or our original hummus. I order the creamy ranch dip. Cherry tomatoes, zucchini slices, sliced red, yellow and green peppers, baby carrots, broccoli crowns, yellow squash, and cauliflower heads.

Fruit – Hand-picked seasonal fresh fruits ripe for the picking. A delightful and healthy option for your next party or meeting.

Condiments – Green leaf lettuce, sliced tomatoes, sliced red onions, sprouts, and pickles. Just the right condiments to accompany our Meat and Cheese Tray, or to complete your next BBQ.

Petite Sandwiches – A delicious platter of mini-sandwiches made with your choice of savory roast beef, turkey breast or chicken salad, all dressed to your liking. Mayonnaise and mustard packets are included.

Croissant Sandwiches – Buttery, flaky mini-croissants topped with your choice of roast beef, turkey or handmade chicken salad, dressed and ready for your guests to enjoy. Mustard and mayonnaise packets are included.

Meat and Cheese Tray – Savory slices of roast beef and turkey combined with fresh slices of cheddar, provolone and Swiss cheese. Includes rolls, mustard and mayonnaise packets.

Gourmet Cheese – Indulge in our finest cheese selections from around the world. Choose from Manchego or Iberico from

Spain, beautiful Brie from France or Jarlsberg from Norway. And don't forget about the incredible selection of cheese from the good ol' USA, like Salemville blue cheese from Wisconsin and Farmstead goat cheeses. If these don't tempt your palate, you are welcome to select your favorites from our cheese tables to customize your tray.

Fruit and Cheese – What goes with cheese? Well, fruit of course! Enjoy both on this delicious tray of cubed domestic cheese, decorated with seasonal fruit. Perfect for snacks or meetings.

Cheese and Nothing but Cheese – A group of classic cheeses like cheddar, Colby Jack, hot pepper Jack and smoked gouda. Perfect for snacking.

Whole Foods Market

Catering Menu
Chain Supermarket

Party Starters:

Mix & Match

Eggrolls & Potstickers – Chose from veggie, chicken, or pork potstickers or split eggrolls. Served with Asian dipping sauce. I order the chicken or veggie and do not use the dipping sauce.

Skewers – Choose from grilled Thai curry chicken, chipotle beef, fresh mozzarella with tomato & basil, or sweet chili tofu. I order the chicken, beef, and mozzarella with tomatoes.

Mini Meatballs – Choose 1 variety of meatball; turkey, buffalo and quinoa, or vegetarian. Choose 1 sauce; marinara, roasted red pepper sauce, artichoke, or herbed tomato sauce. I order the turkey or vegetarian meatballs and one of the sauces

Party Platters:

Deli Sliders – Choice of any 3 of the following: Sonoma chicken salad, classic chicken salad, cranberry tuna, lemon dill tuna, vegetable hummus, curry turkey, or vegan curry chicken salad. I order the Sonoma chicken salad, classic chicken salad, curry turkey, or vegan curry chicken salad. I ask the deli counterperson to leave off the bread.

Antipasti Platter – Prosciutto, salami, tortellini, fresh mozzarella, goat cheese, provolone, artichoke hearts, and kalamata olives served with balsamic vinaigrette. I ask the deli counterperson to give me extra cheese in place of the prosciutto and the tortellini.

Vegetable Crudité Platter – Fresh assortment of crisp, colorful seasonal vegetables served with red pepper ranch dip.

Continental Fruit & Cheese - Fresh fruit paired with cheddar, Jarlsberg, and Havarti.

Asian Cheese Board – A selection of gourmet cheeses including bleu, honey-fig brie, Parrano, goat cheese, and cheddar served with red grapes, almonds, and dried figs. I ask the deli counterperson to substitute strawberries for the red grapes and the dried figs.

Deli Meat & Cheese – A selection of sliced or cubed cheddar, Jarlsberg, Havarti, Black Forest Ham, roasted turkey and roast beef, served with red grapes. I ask the deli counterperson to substitute extra roast beef or turkey for the ham and strawberries for the red grapes.

Specialty Platters:

Build Your Brie – To top our exclusive and most popular brie with your choice of preserves and/or nuts for a decadent appetizer or holiday party treat. Preserve toppings include apricot, cherry, fig, and cranberry. Nut toppings include marcona almonds, caramelized walnuts, pistachios, and caramelized pecans. I do not eat preservatives or caramelized nuts.

Spanish Cheese Platter – Enjoy a taste of Spain's flavors and textures with Manchego, Drunken Goat, Mahon, Capricho de Cabra, and Campo Montalban. Paired with dates and fresh grapes. I ask the deli counterperson to substitute strawberries for the dates and grapes.

Breakfast & Brunch:

Oven-Fresh Quiche – Your choice of quiche Lorraine, broccoli cheese, or spinach mushroom. I order the broccoli cheese or spinach mushroom. I do not eat the crust.

Fresh Fruit and Dip Tray – Fresh seasonal fruit with creamy vanilla dip.

Specialty Salads:

Maple Pecan Cranberry Salad – field greens, feta cheese, dried cranberries, red onions, and cucumbers tossed in vinaigrette then topped with maple-glazed pecans. I ask the deli counterperson to substitute extra field greens for the cucumbers and fresh pecans for the maple-glazed pecans.

Mozzarella, Basil, and Tomato – Fresh handmade mozzarella layered with tomatoes, basil, and balsamic vinaigrette on a bed of field greens.

Strawberry Spinach Salad – Fresh spinach, fresh strawberries, feta cheese, almonds, and orange raspberry vinaigrette.

Field Greens Salad – Fresh field greens, roasted tomatoes, bleu cheese, and walnuts in a balsamic vinaigrette.

HSH Thai Peanut Salad – Shredded green, red, and Napa cabbage, red onions snow peas, edamame, red bell peppers, cilantro, green onions, and toasted peanuts in a sesame ginger dressing. I ask the deli counterperson to substitute extra snow peas for the edamame.

Classic Salads:

Classic Garden Salad - Spring mix and romaine tossed with tomatoes, cucumber, carrots, and red onion. Served with ranch dressing. I ask the deli counterperson to substitute extra tomatoes for the cucumbers.

Caesar Salad – Crispy romaine, tomatoes, and parmesan cheese served with Caesar dressing and topped with freshly made croutons. I ask the deli counterperson to substitute extra romaine for the croutons and to substitute bleu cheese dressing for the Caesar dressing.

Sandwiches & Boxed Lunches:

Build-Your own Sandwich Platter – Sliced roasted turkey, Black Forest ham, roast beef, cheddar, Swiss and provolone cheeses. Includes lettuce, tomatoes, onion, pickles, and condiments. Served with fresh-baked bread. I ask the deli counterperson to substitute extra roast beef for the ham and to substitute extra lettuce, tomatoes, onions, and pickles for the breads.

Entrées:

Grilled Chicken Breast – Chose from classic, rosemary, or bbq. I order the classic or rosemary chicken.

Carne Asada – Simply marinated, grilled, and served with cilantro pesto.

Canadian Steak Seasoned Eye of Round – Marinated, then slow-roasted.

Beef Tenderloin with Garlic and Herbs – Juicy tenderloin of beef prepared medium rare. Sliced thin and served with horseradish sauce.

Prime Rib – Perfectly seasoned and roasted medium rare. Served with au jus and horseradish sauce.

Feasts & Sides:

Fajita or Taco Bar – Choice of seasoned ground beef, chicken, or vegetarian picadillo served with sautéed onions & peppers, lettuce, cheese, tomatoes, sour cream, salsa, and choice of corn or flour tortillas. I ask the deli counterperson to substitute extra lettuce and tomatoes for the corn and flour tortillas and the sour cream.

Mediterranean Bar – hummus, dolmas, olives, feta, falafel, tabbouleh, chicken, lettuce, tomatoes, pickled vegetables, tzatzki Sauce and served with pitas. I ask the deli counterperson to substitute extra pickled vegetables for the tabbouleh and the pita.

Home Style Sides – Grilled, roasted, or steamed vegetable medley.

Sweet Endings:

Using only cage-free eggs.

Chocolate Lover's Dream – An abundantly rich assortment of all chocolate goodies you could hope for: chocolate-covered strawberries, specialty chocolates, and chocolate baked goods.

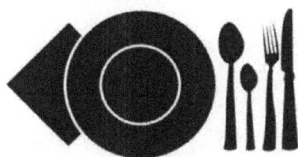

AIRPORT RESTAURANTS

Chili's/Chili's Too

Chain Restaurant

The Chili's Too menu is not listed here because it is listed under Chili's in the first edition of *From Fat to Fabulous: A Diet Guide for Restaurant Lovers*

Rio Grande Brew Pub & Grill

Sunport International Airport
Albuquerque, NM

Sunrise:

Steak and Eggs – An 8 oz. center cut sirloin steak grilled to perfection with two eggs cooked to order and southwestern potatoes and your choice of wheat or white toast. I ask the waitperson to substitute tomato slices for the potatoes.

Egg Whites – Make it a healthier choice, substitute egg whites in your omelet or scrambled eggs.

Breakfast Buffet – Cooked to order omelets, scrambled eggs, fruit, and yogurt.

Appetizers:

Sliders – Your choice of three ground chuck mini cheeseburgers topped with a pickle or our signature brisket chipotle barbeque sliders.

Soups and Salads:

Chef's Daily Soup

Green Chili Soup – A New Mexican favorite. A spicy blend of green chile, potatoes, vegetables and cheese, served with a warm tortilla – named one of USA Today's top soups in the country! I do not eat the tortilla or the potatoes.

The Harvest – Fresh spinach, walnuts, red onions, tomatoes, avocado, and bleu cheese crumbles and a raspberry vinaigrette. For an extra charge add grilled chicken. I add the grilled chicken and ask the waitperson to ask the chef to substitute extra tomatoes for the avocado.

Caesar Salad – Crisp Romaine lettuce tossed in a creamy Caesar dressing topped with seasoned croutons and shredded parmesan cheese. For an extra charge add grilled chicken. I order the grilled chicken and ask the waitperson to ask the chef to substitute extra Romaine lettuce for the croutons and bleu cheese dressing for the Caesar dressing.

Chef Salad - Fresh mixed greens topped with thinly sliced turkey and ham, cheddar cheese, tomatoes, hard-boiled eggs and black olives – served with seasoned croutons and your choice of dressing. I ask the waitperson to ask the chef to substitute extra turkey for the ham and extra mixed greens for the croutons.

Farmer's Salad – Fresh mixed greens, ripe tomatoes, cucumbers, avocado and red onions tossed together with seasoned croutons – served with your choice of dressing. I ask the waitperson to ask the chef to substitute extra tomatoes and onions for the cucumbers, avocado, and croutons.

Dressings – Ranch, bleu cheese, Italian, raspberry vinaigrette.

Burgers and Sandwiches:

Your choice of one side available: steamed veggies.

Rio Grande Chicken – A tender and juicy charbroiled chicken breast on a freshly baked warm bun dressed with mushroom, green chile, and melted Swiss cheese.

Rio Grande Cheeseburger – 8 oz. New Mexico beef patty charbroiled and topped with a crisp, lightly battered green chile, hickory smoked cheddar cheese and chipotle mayo. I ask the waitperson to ask the chef to leave off the batter on the green chile.

BBQ Brisket Sandwich – Smoked tender beef brisket, tossed in our signature BBQ sauce served on a warm, toasted bun.

New Mexico Philly – Thinly sliced roast beef with green chile and melted Swiss cheese on a soft French roll – accompanied by beef au jus for dipping.

Build Your Own Burger – Create your own gastronomic masterpiece on an 8 oz. New Mexico beef patty. Each burger comes garnished with lettuce, tomato, and pickles. For an extra charge you can add green chile, mushrooms, cheddar cheese, bleu cheese crumbles, pepper Jack or Swiss.

Entrées:

Available Sides: steamed vegetable medley.

Southwestern Ribeye – 10 oz. hand crafted choice Ribeye steak charbroiled to perfection and served with your choice of two sides and a dinner roll.

Petit Filet – A 6 oz. hand crafted choice tenderloin, cooked to your liking with your choice of two sides and a dinner roll.

Desserts:

Almond Tart – Homemade and served to you warm.

Rio Grande Rootbeer Float – Rio Grande's signature draft rootbeer poured over scoops of vanilla ice cream in a frost y mug.

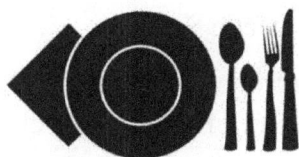

HOTEL DINING

Marriott

Cielo Sandia
Hotel Chain

Begin:

Thai Spring Rolls – Chicken, Napa slaw, orange ginger sauce and sriracha aioli.

Warmth:

Today's Freshly Made Soup.

Chicken Tortilla Soup – Tortilla chips. I ask the waitperson to ask the chef to leave off the tortilla chips.

Three Cheese Onion Grantinee – Gruyere, provolone, and parmesan. I ask the waitperson to ask the chef to leave off the bread or croutons.

Greens:

Caesar Salad – Grilled rosemary chicken, shaved parmesan cheese. I ask the waitperson to ask the chef to leave off the croutons and to substitute bleu cheese for the Caesar dressing.

Asian Chicken Salad – Grilled spicy chicken, cucumber sticks, tomatoes, carrots, almonds, and mandarin dressing. I ask the waitperson to ask the chef to substitute extra tomatoes for the cucumber sticks.

Sandwich & Soup:

Your choice of sandwich with soup selection or side salad.

Breads:

Served with French fries or house-made kettle chips. On all sandwiches I ask the waitperson to ask the chef to substitute a small salad or a vegetable for the fries or chips.

Reuben – Slow simmered corned beef brisket, Swiss cheese, sauerkraut, 1000 Island dressing on grilled rye bread. I ask the waitperson to ask the chef to substitute yellow mustard for the 1000 Island dressing.

Philly Cheese Steak – Shaved rib eye, mushrooms, onions, banana peppers, provolone on a baguette.

Cali Chicken – Grilled chicken, hardwood bacon, avocado, Swiss cheese, Bibb lettuce and tomato. I ask the waitperson to ask the chef to substitute extra tomato and lettuce for the bacon and avocado.

Chipotle Chicken Wrap – Grilled chicken, guacamole, Pico de Gallo, Jack and cheddar, sun-dried tomato wrap. I ask the waitperson to ask the chef to substitute extra cheddar cheese for the guacamole.

BBQ Brisket – Slow roasted brisket, sweet BBQ sauce, brioche roll and Napa slaw. I ask the waitperson to ask the chef to substitute mustard for the sweet BBQ sauce.

Burger Bar:

Angus Burger with Cheese – Selection of cheese, Bibb lettuce, tomato, sweet onion on a brioche roll.

Angus Blue Mushroom Burger – Sautéed mushrooms, blue cheese, Bibb lettuce, tomato, sweet onion on a brioche roll.

Turkey Burger – Lean ground turkey seared, Bibb lettuce, tomato, brioche roll and fat free mayonnaise on the side.

After 5 Selections:

Served with Yukon gold mashed, unless specified. Add a house salad or a Caesar for an additional charge. On all dishes I ask the waitperson to ask the chef to substitute the house salad or a vegetable for the Yukon gold mashed potatoes.

Stock Yards® Angus Beef Rib Eye – Grilled center cut rib eye, red wine dimi and roasted Brussels sprouts.

Stock Yards® Angus Beef Filet – Grilled filet mignon, red wine demi and roasted Brussels sprouts.

<u>Chicken Gran Mere</u> – Roasted chicken breast, sautéed mushrooms, hardwood bacon, caramelized onion, sautéed broccolini. I ask the waitperson to ask the chef to substitute extra broccolini for the bacon.

<u>Papardelle Barolo</u> – Shaved boneless short rib, Barolo wine glace, fresh herbs finished with horseradish cream.

<u>Brisket of Beef</u> – Slow smoked BBQ brisket, Yukon gold mashed and roasted Brussels sprouts. I ask the waitperson to ask the chef to substitute broccolini for the mashed potatoes.

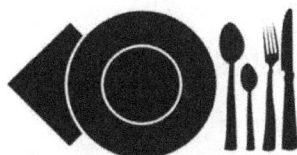

WHOLESALE/FOOD WAREHOUSES

Costco

Chain Wholesaler

Fresh:

Fresh fruits and vegetables.

Drinks:

Bottled water.

Tea.

Prepared & Packaged Food:

Ann's House Unsalted Cashews.

Kirkland Signature Extra Fancy Unsalted Mixed Nuts – Cashews, Pistachios, Almonds, and Pecans.

Cello Variety Pack Premium Sliced Cheeses – Aged Cheddar, French Swiss, Creamy Havarti, and Dutch Gouda.

Burgers By Amylu - Sweet caramelized onion chicken burgers with red bell peppers and Gouda cheese.

Chef Bruce Aidells Chicken Meatballs with Teriyaki & Pineapple – Teriyaki Chicken meatballs with pineapple and garlic.

Cuisine Solutions All Natural 2 Lamb Shanks Fully Cooked – Savory seasoned lamb in a Portobello mushroom and red wine sauce.

Morton's of Omaha Beef Pot Roast with Gravy – Made with natural beef juices.

Saffron Road Lamb Saag – Lambs raised without antibiotics. Tender lamb cubes lightly spiced with Turmeric and authentic herbs. Served with a thick bed of spinach.

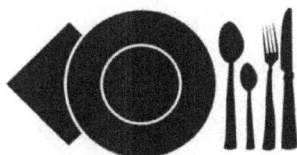

RESTAURANTS RAISING FUNDS FOR CHARITABLE CAUSES

The Woman's Exchange

St. Louis, MO
Established 1883

Tea Room Hours – 11:15 A.M. -2:30 PM Monday - Saturday

The Woman's Exchange of St. Louis is a volunteer, not-for-profit organization dedicated to the principle of helping those in need to lead productive lives by earning a living through their talents and the sale of their unique handmade merchandise. The Exchange fosters a sense of pride, involvement, and mutual support through sustained and varied opportunities to achieve an improved quality of life.

The Woman's Exchange Sandwiches:

Served on fresh white, whole wheat, marble rye, 15 grain, sourdough, or chose a spinach tortilla wrap. Served with sweet pickles and your choice of side: fresh fruit or cottage cheese.

Country Club Sandwich – Sliced chicken breast, ham, crisp bacon, garden fresh lettuce, tomato, onion, smoked cheddar cheese with honey mustard. I ask the waitperson to ask the chef to substitute extra chicken for the ham and extra tomato for the bacon.

Classic Club Sandwich – Served with chicken breast, crisp bacon, tomato, garden fresh lettuce and mayonnaise. I ask the waitperson to ask the chef to substitute extra tomato for the bacon.

Veggie Sandwich – The Exchange's combination of tomato, lettuce, red onion, cucumbers, and Havarti cheese served with the Exchange's House Dressing. I ask the waitperson to ask the chef to substitute extra tomato for the cucumbers.

Café Sandwiches – Choice of sliced chicken breast, house-made chicken salad, or egg salad served with garden fresh lettuce.

The Euclid Avenue – An open faced sandwich of sliced

tomatoes and crisp bacon smothered in the Exchange's secret cheddar cheese spread then broiled to golden perfection. I ask the waitperson to ask the chef to substitute extra chicken for the bacon.

The Maryland Ave. – The Exchange's classic combination of cream cheese and green olives grilled on your choice of bread.

The W. E. Wrap – Enjoy the Woman's Exchange salad in a spinach tortilla.

The Celebration Wrap – Chicken salad, crispy bacon, lettuce, tomato, and the Exchange's House Dressing wrapped in a spinach tortilla. I ask the waitperson to ask the chef to substitute extra tomato for the bacon.

The Asparagus Melt – Blanched asparagus and thinly sliced ham served open-faced, topped with melted parmesan-goat cheese spread. I ask the waitperson to ask the chef to substitute extra chicken for the ham.

Classic Hamburger – The traditional American favorite served with lettuce, tomato, red onion, and dill pickles.

For an additional charge add your choice of cheese – cheddar, pepper jack, smoked Gouda, dill Havarti, or mozzarella.

The Woman's Exchange Salads & Plates:

Each salad is served with your choice of dressing and a toasted English muffin. I do not eat the English muffin. Salads are available full or half size.

The Famous Woman's Exchange Salad – Fresh chicken breast, ham Swiss cheese, tomato, hard-boiled egg, crisp bacon, green onion, and garden fresh lettuce, hand-chopped and served with the Exchange's House Dressing. I ask the waitperson to ask the chef to substitute extra chicken for the ham and to substitute extra lettuce for the bacon.

Strawberry Spinach Salad – Fresh spinach, sliced strawberries, toasted almonds, chopped red onion, crisp bacon, and feta cheese, served with poppy seed dressing. I ask the waitperson to ask the chef to substitute extra spinach for the bacon.

"The Diet" Salad – A medley of chicken, tomatoes, green onions, and chopped garden fresh lettuce served with your choice of dressing.

Tossed Green Salad – A medley of tomatoes, green onions, hard-boiled eggs, olives, cucumbers, and garden fresh lettuce with the Exchange's House Dressing. I ask the waitperson to ask the chef to substitute extra green onions for the cucumbers.

Dressing Choices – The Woman's Exchange House Dressing, Honey Mustard, French, and Fat Free Raspberry Vinaigrette.

Café Salad Plates:

Your choice of house-made chicken salad, egg salad, or cottage cheese served on a bed of garden fresh lettuce, surrounded by fresh fruit or veggies.

The Salad Trio Plate – Your choice of three petite scoops: chicken salad, egg salad, or cottage cheese surrounded by fresh fruit or veggies.

Protein Plate – Hamburger patty served with cottage cheese and sliced tomato on a bed of lettuce.

Diet Plate – Sliced chicken and tomatoes on a bed of lettuce.

A Little of Everything:

Pick Two Favorites – Cup of the Exchange's soup du jour, half a sandwich of your choice (sliced chicken, chicken salad, or egg salad), or Petite Woman's Exchange Salad.

Soup Du Jour:

The Exchange's hot and delicious soups, prepared daily in our kitchen. Cup, bowl, pint, or quart.

Children's Specials:

All are served with potato chips and sweet pickles. I ask the waitperson to ask the chef to substitute fruit for the potato chips.

Hamburger – cheese is an additional charge.

Just Desserts:

Signature Coconut Cake

A Selection of Pies

Chocolate Mint Brownies

A Selection of Cookies

A catering and box lunch menu are also available.

HE FIRST AND SECOND EDITION of the highly acclaimed *FROM FAT TO FABULOUS: A DIET GUIDE FOR RESTAURANT LOVERS* is available in paperback or as an eBook. They are available online or your favorite bookseller can order it for you.

THURSDAY'S CHILD and *ANOTHER THURSDAY'S CHILD,* the award-winning nonfiction short story series, are also available in paperback and as an eBook. They are available online or your favorite bookseller can order them for you.

Look for **RED CARPET PRESS** fantastic books online or order them from your favorite bookseller.

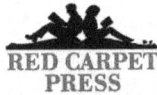

RED CARPET PRESS

"Rolling Out the 'Read' Carpet, One Fantastic Book at a Time.™"

ABOUT THE AUTHOR, E. S. ABRAMSON

ELAINE SANDRA ABRAMSON, writing as E. S. Abramson, is an award-winning artist and author. She is the first woman State Artist of Texas. Her artwork and writing have been on TV, the Internet, used in Texas tourism, and on licensed merchandise.

She worked with Viacom Entertainment and the Pixelon Network, and is a former director of the Animagic International Animation Studio School.

She created the "Creative Entrepreneur Workshops" for artists and authors for Richland College, and gives workshops around the country.

Ms. Abramson, her husband, and their Labrador retriever live in St. Louis and Albuquerque.

Visit our website at www.Red-Carpet-Press.com.

Visit the author's website at www.ElaineAbramson.com.

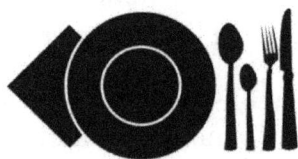

Visit

**Red Carpet Press online at
www.Red-Carpet-Press.com**

Keep up on our latest new
releases from your favorite
authors, as well as author
appearances, news, blogs,
chats, special offers and
more.

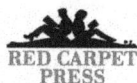

RED CARPET
PRESS

"Rolling Out the 'Read' Carpet, One Fantastic Book at a Time.™"

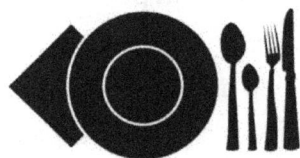

www.ingramcontent.com/pod-product-compliance
Lightning Source LLC
Chambersburg PA
CBHW031148270326
41931CB00006B/191